Anuj Mansata
Neelampari Parikh
C. Nandini

Tumour Immunology

Anuj Mansata
Neelampari Parikh
C. Nandini

Tumour Immunology

An insight to complex mechanisms of tumour
growth

LAP LAMBERT Academic Publishing

Imprint

Any brand names and product names mentioned in this book are subject to trademark, brand or patent protection and are trademarks or registered trademarks of their respective holders. The use of brand names, product names, common names, trade names, product descriptions etc. even without a particular marking in this work is in no way to be construed to mean that such names may be regarded as unrestricted in respect of trademark and brand protection legislation and could thus be used by anyone.

Cover image: www.ingimage.com

Publisher:
LAP LAMBERT Academic Publishing
is a trademark of
Dodo Books Indian Ocean Ltd. and OmniScriptum S.R.L publishing group

120 High Road, East Finchley, London, N2 9ED, United Kingdom
Str. Armeneasca 28/1, office 1, Chisinau MD-2012, Republic of Moldova, Europe
Managing Directors: Ieva Konstantinova, Victoria Ursu
info@omniscriptum.com

Printed at: see last page
ISBN: 978-3-659-78498-9

CONTENTS

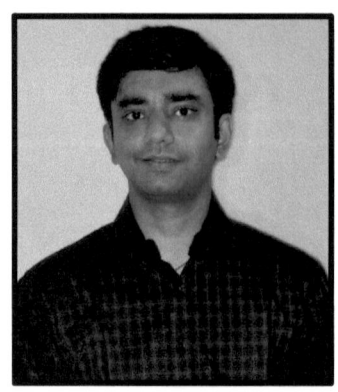

Dedicated to

My Grandfather

Late L. N. Mansata

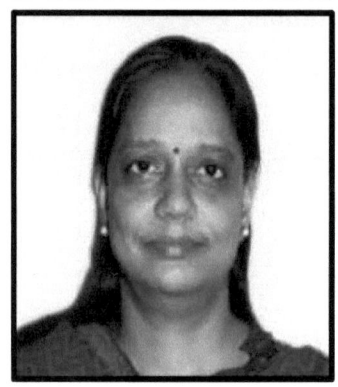

Dedicated to

My Parents

Late Nirmalaben Parikh &

Rajendra Parikh,

My brother

Paras R. Parikh &

My niece - Vishva

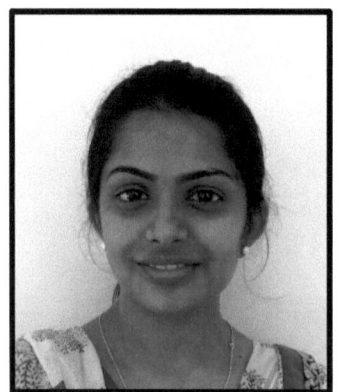

Dedicated to

My Family

[2]

1. <u>INTRODUCTION:</u>

CANCER is derived from Latin word for Crab – that is, they adhere to any part that they seize in an obstinate manner, similar to a crab's behaviour.[1] Cancer is a collective term for a disease induced by multicausal changes of the genetic information i.e. Deoxyribonucleic acid (DNA) of the cell. The genetic changes result in an unregulated proliferation of these cells and their descendants. In tumour cells a continuous randomized loss and gain of DNA takes place, a process known as genetic instability. This genetic instability results in an inexhaustible source of new and altered proteins, which may be recognized by the immune system.

Cancer is the second leading cause of death in the world after cardiovascular diseases. Appearance of a tumour (from the Latin word for "swelling") results from ABNORMAL PROLIFERATION of cells, through the loss or modification of normal growth control. Cells which normally do not divide (e.g. muscle or kidney cells) may start proliferating, or cells which normally do proliferate (e.g. basal epithelial cells or hemopoeitic cells) may begin dividing in an uncontrolled fashion. If the growth of a tumour remains localized, it can often be removed surgically (if it is accessible), and is therefore relatively harmless; or "benign". In some cases, however, cells from a growing tumour may be capable of intruding into adjacent normal tissue ("invasive growth"), and may leave the original site and begin to proliferate in a new location (METASTASIS). These properties distinguish "MALIGNANT" tumours from benign ones.[2]

<u>CONVENTIONAL MODES OF TREATMENT:</u>

The immune system has evolved in order to detect and eliminate the pathogens that may do harm to the organism. It serves as a watchdog against transformed cells that may lead to cancer. [3]

Surgery, chemotherapy, radiation therapy, etc are the conventional methods of treating cancer. However surgery involving radical dissections causes severe debilitation to the patient. Chemotherapy and Radiotherapy also have dangerous side effects leading to harm to the normal tissue along with the tumour. Considering these ill effects, newer modes of cancer treatment are being researched since last few decades. Immune system of the body is found to have role in tumour pathogenesis. Scientists like Paul Ehrlich, Burnet, and Macfarlane studied the tumour immunology and found evidences supporting role of immune system.

EVIDENCE OF TUMOR IMMUNITY:

- Spontaneous regression: melanoma, lymphoma
- Regression of metastases after removal of primary tumor: pulmonary metastases from renal carcinoma
- Infiltration of tumors by lymphocytes and macrophages: melanoma and breast cancer
- Lymphocyte proliferation in draining lymph nodes
- Higher incidence of cancer after immune-suppression, immunodeficiency (AIDS, neonates), aging, etc.

HISTORY OF RESEARCH IN TUMOR IMMUNOLOGY:

In 1909, Paul Ehrlich predicted that the immune system repressed the growth of carcinomas that he envisaged would otherwise occur with great frequency (Ehrlich, 1909), thus initiating a century of contentious debate over immunologic control of neoplasia. Fifty years later as immunologists gained an enhanced understanding of transplantation and tumour immune-biology and immune-genetics, F. Macfarlane Burnet and Lewis Thomas revisited the topic of natural immune protection against cancer. Burnet's thinking was shaped by a consideration of immune tolerance; he believed that tumour cell-specific neo-antigens could provoke an effective

[4]

immunologic reaction that would eliminate developing cancers (Burnet, 1957, 1964, 1971). Alternatively, Thomas's early view was evolutionary in nature; he theorized that complex long-lived organisms must possess mechanisms to protect against neoplastic disease similar to that mediating homograft rejection (Thomas, 1959).[4]

With the functional demonstration of mouse tumour-specific antigens supporting the ideas of Ehrlich, Burnet, and Thomas (Old and Boyse, 1964), the cancer immune-surveillance hypothesis, which stated that sentinel thymus dependent cells of the body constantly surveyed host tissues for nascently transformed cells (Burnet, 1970), gained recognition. Despite subsequent challenges to this hypothesis over the next several decades (Stutman 1974, 1979), new studies in the 1990s—fueled by technologic advances in mouse genetics and monoclonal antibody (mAb) production—reinvigorated and ultimately validated the cancer immune-surveillance concept (Smyth et al., 2001b; Dunn et al., 2002, 2004) and expanded it to incorporate the contributions of both innate and adaptive immunity.[4]

Two different models for the immune response to tumours have been proposed: the concept of immunosurveillance and the danger model. According to the immunosurveillance hypothesis, tumours expressing antigens are regarded as "nonself" by the immune system, and a major function of the immune system is to survey the body for the development of malignancy and to eliminate tumour cells as they arise [8]. To detect "danger," the immune system uses professional antigen-presenting cells (APC) as sentinels of tissue damage. In the presence of danger signals, APC—such as dendritic cells, activated macrophages, and B cells—stimulate the T cell response. The danger model proposes that cancer cells do not appear dangerous to the immune system, so that the response of T cells to tumours is not initiated. [5]

Since the evaluation of cancer in immune-suppressed patients – in those with transplantations in whom immunosuppressive drugs were used, with acquired immune deficiency syndrome or congenital immune deficiency diseases – the importance of the immune system in the initial prevention of cancer has become clear. The incidence of most common forms of cancer in immune suppressed patients is no different from that in the general population. However, some virally induced cancers, such as Epstein–Barr virus (EBV)-induced B-cell lymphoma, are significantly increased in immune deficient patients. Notably not the infection but the development of malignant clones from the latently infected B cells is prevented by the immune system. There is also an increase in other virus associated malignancies such as Human papilloma virus (HPV)-induced cervical carcinoma and Hepatitis B virus induced hepatocellular carcinoma. [2]

The main indicator of cancer is the uncontrolled growth and dispersion of cells as a result of abnormal changes to the genetic material contained in those cells. A single cell or group of cells can undergo genetic events such as mutations, influenced by inherited or environmental factors as well as a result of certain levels of hormones or growth factors, which may change the cells' behaviours. These events, which may take years to arise, cause the cells to proceed down the pathway to the development of cancer. [6]

If cells divide abnormally in an early stage of development, they may evolve into a cell population that could be immortalized and which may lose the control mechanisms of normal cell division, activity and interactions with neighbouring cells. Such immortalized cell populations may evolve into malignant tumour cell populations, whose behaviour may violate the tissue environment. [6]

Once certain cell populations become malignant they may form solid tumours which invade and destroy same tissues as well as they may metastasize (spread) all over the body by releasing tumour cells into the blood and lymph system, where they may continue to grow and develop by forming new cancers. [6]

Tumour immunotherapy makes use of biological agents that mimic some of the natural signals that body uses to control tumour growth. These natural biological agents can now be produced in the laboratory including interferons, interleukins, cytokines, endogenous angio-inhibitors and antigens.

In 1990s scientists produced therapeutic monoclonal antibodies rituximab and trastuzumab that specifically targeted lymphoma and breast cancer cells. At present scientists are developing vaccines to boost the body's immune response against cancer cells.[7]Until late 1990's most of the drugs used in cancer therapy worked by killing cancer cells. Unfortunately chemotherapy agents used, also killed some normal cells and had a greater effect on cancer cells.[7]

During the past two decades, the paradigm for cancer treatment has evolved from relatively nonspecific cytotoxic agents to selective, mechanism-based therapeutics. Cancer chemotherapies were initially identified through screens for compounds that killed rapidly dividing cells. These drugs remain the backbone of current treatment, but they are limited by a narrow therapeutic index, significant toxicities and frequently acquired resistance. More recently, an improved understanding of cancer pathogenesis has given rise to new treatment options, including targeted agents and cancer immunotherapy. [8]

The study of immunotherapy in cancer spans several decades with hundreds of clinical trials, using many different immune-stimulatory strategies and modalities for vaccine delivery. A wealth of knowledge is now available that suggests that immunotherapy has potential application in the treatment of cancer, where it has been demonstrated to induce both clinical responses and robust immunological responses in sub-groups of treated patients.[9]

Advantages of immunotherapy:
- Stimulates body's own immune system to fight the disease.

- Tumour-specific Immune Response.
- Relatively less side effects as compared to chemotherapy and surgical as well as radiotherapy.

Interactions between the immune system and malignant cells play an important role in tumorigenesis. Failure of the immune system to detect and reject transformed cells may lead to cancer development. Tumours use multiple mechanisms to escape from immune-mediated rejection. Many of these mechanisms are now known on a cellular and molecular level.[5]

This work is an attempt to review the basic immunology, the role of immune involvement in the prevention or cure of human cancers and an insight into the advances in the field of tumour immunology and immunotherapy.

2. BASIC IMMUNOLOGY:

The meaning of the word immunity derives from the Latin word immunis (unhurt, protected) and describes the protection and immunity against particular infectious agents. The term "immunity" has traditionally referred to the resistance exhibited by the host towards injury caused by microorganisms and their products. During the encounter with foreign microorganisms the immune system runs through a learn process whereby the recognition of the infectious agents is a crucial step in immune defence. Immunity against infectious disease is of different types.

Innate Native Immunity	Acquired (Adaptive) Immunity
(a) Nonspecific	(a) Active
(b) Specific	(b) Passive

Innate or native immunity is the resistance to infections that an individual possesses by virtue of his or her genetic and constitutional make-up. It is not affected by prior contact with microorganisms or immunisation. It may be non-specific, when it indicates a degree of resistance to infections in general, or specific where resistance to a particular pathogen is concerned.

The adaptive immune system consists of lymphocytes and their products, including antibodies. The receptors of lymphocytes are much more diverse than those of the innate immune system, but lymphocytes are not inherently specific for microbes, and they are capable of recognizing a vast array of foreign substances. There are two types of adaptive immunity: humoral immunity, which protects against extracellular microbes and their toxins, and cell-mediated (or cellular) immunity, which is responsible for defence against intracellular microbes. Humoral immunity is mediated by B (bone marrow–derived) lymphocytes and their secreted products, antibodies (also called immunoglobulins, Ig), and cellular immunity is mediated by T (thymus-derived) lymphocytes. Both classes of lymphocytes express highly specific receptors for a wide variety of substances, called antigens.[10]

MECHANISMS OF INNATE IMMUNITY:

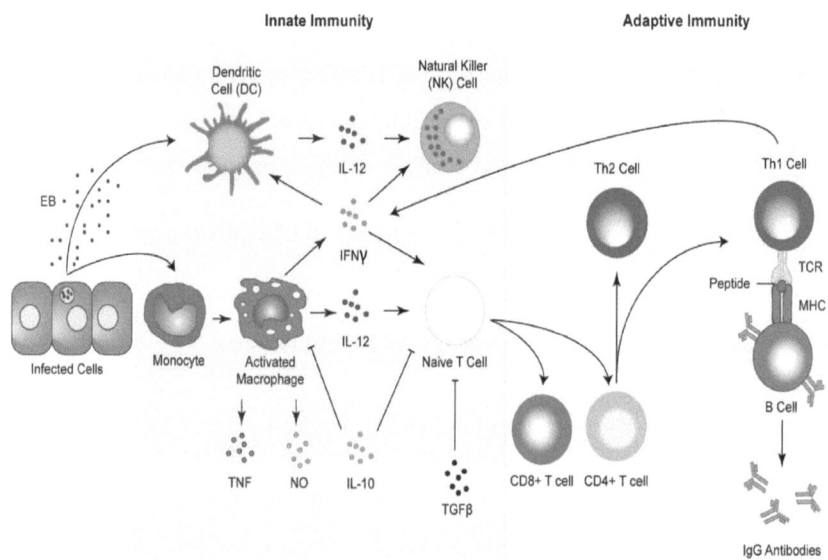

FIGURE 1: TYPES OF IMMUNITY (From Redgrove KA and McLaughlin EA, 2014)

The major components of innate immunity are epithelial barriers that block entry of microbes, phagocytic cells (mainly neutrophils and macrophages), dendritic cells, natural killer (NK) cells, and several plasma proteins, including the proteins of the complement system. The two most important cellular reactions of innate immunity are: inflammation, the process in which phagocytic leukocytes are recruited and activated to kill microbes, and anti-viral defence, mediated by dendritic cells and NK cells.

Leukocytes and epithelial cells that participate in innate immunity are capable of recognizing components of microbes that are shared among related microbes and are often essential for the infectivity of these pathogens (and thus cannot be mutated to allow the microbes to evade the defence mechanisms). These microbial structures are called pathogen associated molecular patterns. Leukocytes also recognize molecules released by injured and necrotic cells, which are sometimes called danger associated molecular patterns. The cellular receptors that recognize these molecules are often called pattern recognition receptors. The best-defined pattern recognition receptors are a family of proteins called Toll-like receptors (TLRs) that are homologous to the Drosophila protein Toll.

THE CELLS & SOLUBLE MEDIATORS OF THE IMMUNE SYSTEM:

Immune responses are mediated by:

1. A variety of cells; &
2. The soluble mediators that these cells secrete.

The leukocytes are central to all immune responses; other cells in the tissues also participate, by signalling to the lymphocytes and responding to the cytokines released by T cells and macrophages.[10]

Immune Cell Generation

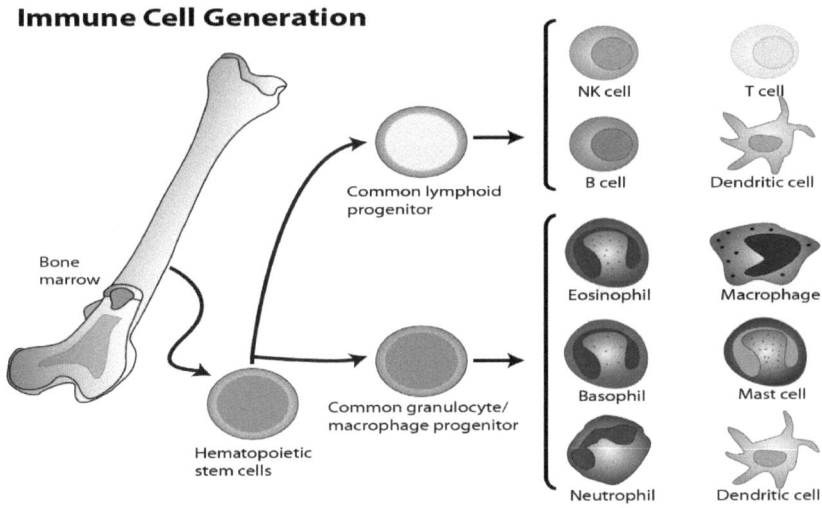

FIGURE 2: COMPONENTS OF THE IMMUNE SYSTEM (From Mary E. Morgan)

PHAGOCYTES:

The most important long-lived phagocytic cells belong to the mononuclear phagocyte lineage. These cells are all derived from bone marrow stem cells, and their function is to:

- engulf particles, including infectious agents;
- internalize them; and
- destroy them.

Leukocytes of the mononuclear phagocyte lineage are called monocytes. Monocytes migrate from the blood into the tissues, where they develop into tissue macrophages, which are very effective at presenting antigens to T cells. Polymorphonuclear neutrophils (often just called neutrophils or PMNs) are another important group of phagocytes. Neutrophils constitute the majority of the blood leukocytes and develop from the same early precursors as monocytes and macrophages. Like monocytes, neutrophils migrate into tissues, particularly at sites of inflammation. Neutrophils are short-lived cells that phagocytose material, destroy it, and then die.

LYMPHOCYTES:

Lymphocytes initiate adaptive immune responses and are wholly responsible for the specific immune recognition of pathogens. In adult mammals, all lymphocytes are derived from bone marrow stem cells, but T lymphocytes (T cells) then develop in the thymus, while B lymphocytes (B cells) develop in the bone marrow.

Different types of T cells have variety of functions.

- Type 1 Helper T cells or TH1 cells: interacts with mononuclear phagocytes and helps them destroy intracellular pathogens.

- Type 2 Helper T cells or TH2: interacts with B cells and helps them to divide, differentiate, and make antibody.

[12]

Cytotoxic T cells (CTLs or Tc cells): Responsible for destruction of host cells that have become infected by viruses or other intracellular pathogens.

T cells recognize antigens present on the surface of other cells using a specific receptor – the T cell antigen receptor (TCR) – which is quite distinct from the antigen receptor (antibody) on B cells.

T cells generate their effects either:

- By releasing soluble proteins, called cytokines, which signal to other cells; or
- By direct cell–cell interactions.

Each B cell is genetically programmed to express a surface receptor specific for a particular antigen. This antigen receptor molecule is called an antibody. If a B cell binds to its specific antigen, it will multiply and differentiate into plasma cells, which produce large amounts of the antibody, but in a secreted form. Secreted antibody molecules are large glycoproteins found in the blood and tissue fluids. Because secreted antibody molecules are a soluble version of the original receptor molecule (antibody), they bind to the same antigen that initially activated the B cells.

CYTOTOXIC CELLS:

Several cell types have the capacity to kill other infected cells. These cells include CTLs, natural killer (NK) cells (large granular lymphocytes) and eosinophils. All of these cell types damage their different targets by releasing the contents of their intracellular granules close to them. Cytokines secreted by the cytotoxic cells, but not stored in granules, contribute to the damage. NK (Natural Killer) cells; also known as Large Granular Lymphocytes (LGLs), have the capacity to recognise the surface changes that occur on a variety of tumour cells and virally infected cells (figure 3). NK cells damage these target cells but use a different recognition system to CTLs. This action is sometimes called NK cell activity, so these cells are also called NK cells. Eosinophils have the ability to engage and damage large extracellular parasites.

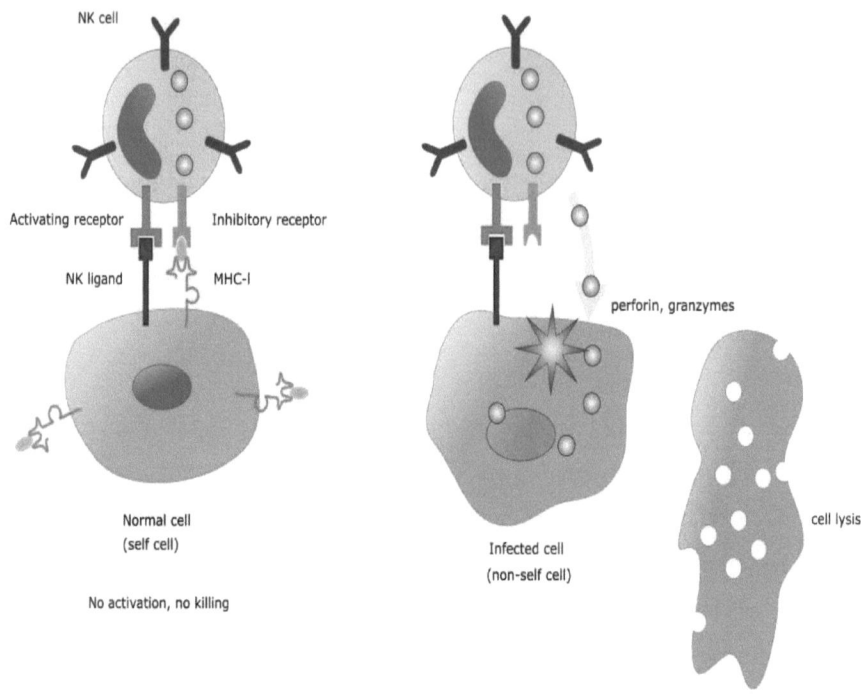

FIGURE 3: NK CELL – MECHANISM OF ACTION (From: www.immuno-oncologynews.com, Patricia Inacio)

AUXILLARY CELLS:

Auxillary cells control inflammation. Inflammation attracts leukocytes and the soluble mediators of immunity towards a site of infection. Mediators of inflammation are released by Basophils, Mast cells and Platelets. Basophils and mast cells have granules that contain a variety of mediators, which:

- Induce inflammation in surrounding tissues; and
- Are released when the cells are triggered.

Basophils and mast cells can also synthesize and secrete a number of mediators that control the development of immune reactions. Mast cells lie close to the blood vessels in all tissues whereas basophils are mobile circulating cells. Platelets play an active role in blood clotting but can be activated during immune response to release mediators of inflammation.

SOLUBLE MEDIATORS OF IMMUNITY:

Antibodies and cytokines produced by lymphocytes and other molecules that are normally present in the serum, constitute the wide variety of molecules that are involved in the development of immune responses. They are also called as Acute Phase Proteins as the serum concentration of a number of these proteins increases rapidly during infection. C-reactive protein (CRP) is an example of Acute phase protein, because of its ability to bind to the C-protein of pneumococci and promotes its Opsonisation i.e. uptake of pneumococci by phagocytes. CRP and complement proteins facilitate protein-coating of bacteria to enhance its phagocytosis and are called Opsonins.

COMPLEMENT:

The complement system is a group of about 20 serum proteins whose overall function is the control of inflammation. The components interact with each other, and with other elements of the immune system. Complement activation is a cascade reaction, where one component acts enzymatically on the next component in the cascade to generate an enzyme, which mediates the next step in the reaction sequence, and so on. The protein molecules or the peptide fragments generated as a result of the activation of the complement system have the following effects (figure 4).

- Attraction of phagocytes to sites of infection (Chemotaxis)
- Opsonisation of microorganisms for uptake by phagocytes and eventual intracellular killing.
- Release of inflammatory mediators from mast cells.

- Increased blood flow to the site of activation and increased permeability of capillaries to plasma molecules.

- Damage to plasma membranes on cells, gram negative bacteria, enveloped viruses or other organisms that have induced the activation, which in turn can result in the lysis of the cell or virus and so reduce the infection.

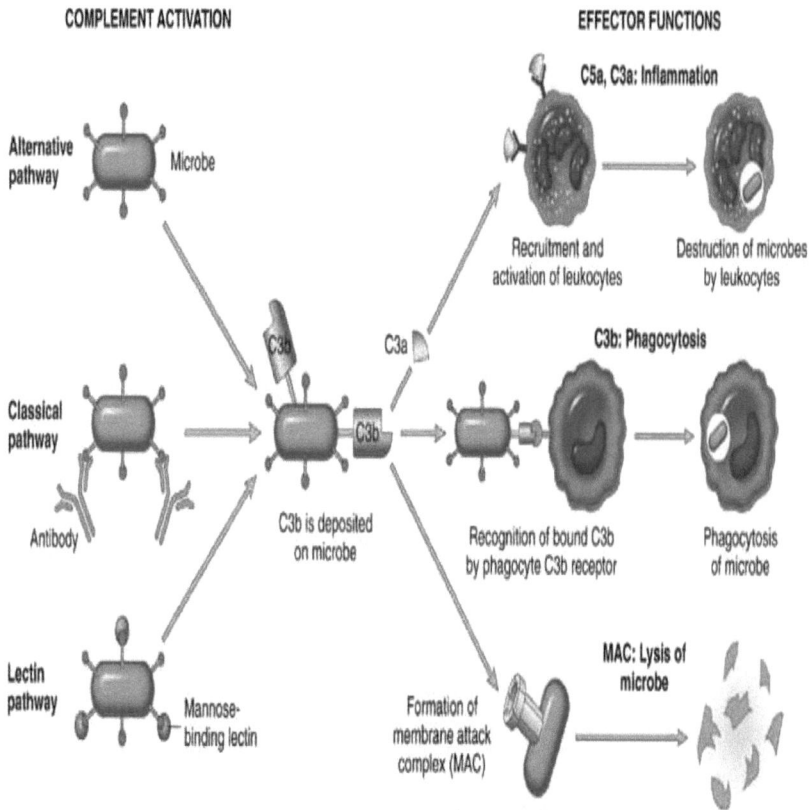

FIGURE 4: FUNCTIONS OF COMPLEMENT (From: Kumar et al. Robbins & Cotran Pathologic Basis of Disease, 8th Edition)

Complement system acts by two pathways:

- A number of microorganisms spontaneously activate the complement system, via the so-called 'alternative pathway', which is an innate immune defence – it results in the microorganism being opsonised (i.e. coated by complement molecules, leading to its uptake by phagocytes).

- The complement system can also be activated by antibodies or by mannose binding lectin bound to the pathogen surface via the 'classical pathway'.

CYTOKINES:

Cytokines are large group of molecules; mostly proteins or glycoproteins, which are involved in signalling between cells during immune responses.[10] Cytokines also maintain the normal growth, migration and survival of immune cells in a physiologic state. Chemokines, interleukins and growth factors are subfamilies of the cytokine family. Cytokines have several important characteristics:

- The same cytokine may be made by a number of different cells.
- The same cytokine may have different effects in different circumstances (this is called 'pleotropy')
- Different cytokines may have the same activity depending on the situation ('redundancy').
- Cytokines often act together and increase the effects of one another ('synergy'). They may also act as antagonists.
- Most cytokines have either paracrine or autocrine effects. Paracrine means they act on cells near to them or that they are actually touching. The autocrine function of IL-2 is well known because, when a T cell is stimulated to make IL-2, it stimulates itself via the IL-2 receptor to proliferate. An example of an uncommon endocrine function for cytokines is IL-1 which can cause fever by stimulating thehypothalamus.[10]

INTERFERONS:

Interferons (IFNs) are cytokines that are particularly important in limiting the spread of certain viral infections:

- One group of interferons (IFNα and IFNβ) is produced by cells that have become infected by a virus;
- Another type, IFNγ, is released by activated TH1 cells.

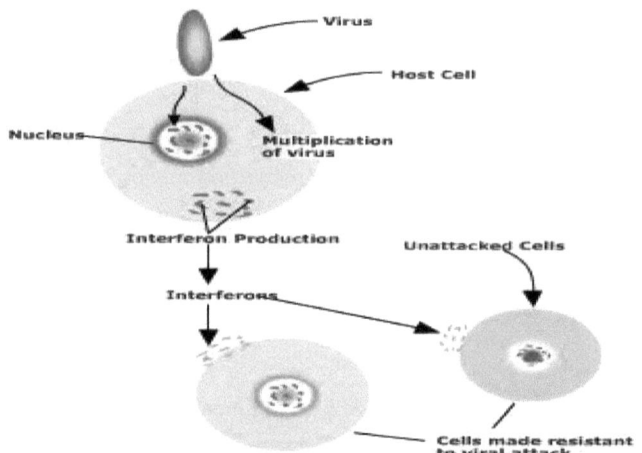

FIGURE 5: INTERFERONS (From: www.tutorvista.com/content/biology/immunity)

IFNs induce a state of antiviral resistance in uninfected cells (figure 5). They are produced very early in infection and are important in delaying the spread of a virus until such time as the adaptive immune response has developed.

INTERLEUKINS:

The interleukins (ILs) are a large group of cytokines produced mainly by T cells, and some are produced by mononuclear phagocytes or by tissue cells. They have a variety of functions. Many interleukins cause other cells to divide and differentiate.

COLONY STIMULATING FACTORS:

Colony stimulating factors (CSFs) are cytokines primarily involved in directing the division and differentiation of bone marrow stem cells, and the precursors of blood leukocytes. The balance of different CSFs is partially responsible for the proportions of different immune cell types produced. Macrophage CSF (M-CSF) promotes the development of monocytes in the bone marrow and macrophages in tissues.

CHEMOKINES:

Chemokines are a large group of chemotactic cytokines that direct the movement of leukocytes around the body, from the blood stream into the tissues and to the appropriate location within each tissue. Some chemokines also activate cells to carry out particular functions.

Other Cytokines include TNF-α & TNF-ß, and TGF-ß – Tumour necrosis factors TNF-α & TNF-ß, and transforming growth factor-ß (TGF-ß), have a variety of functions, but are particularly important in mediating inflammation and cytotoxic reactions.[10]

ANTIGENS:

The term literally means molecules that will generate an antibody response. These molecules are often derived from infectious agents. The pathogen itself is not an antigen; the proteins and carbohydrates that make up the pathogen are antigens. A given pathogen could have thousands of molecules that would be recognized as foreign antigens by the immune system. These antigen molecules are recognized by the immune system by B cells and T cells because they have specific receptors on their surface.

Antigens are not restricted to infectious agents. Tumours often contain modified proteins or proteins not normally expressed which are seen by the immune system as antigens. In autoimmune disease the immune system recognizes normal molecules on the surface of cells as being antigens and these cells are attacked.

It is important to recognize that bacteria or viruses are not themselves antigens but they contain antigens both on their surface and inside them. Such antigens can be isolated and used to safely vaccinate against infection by the whole organism. It is also important to recognize that the T cell receptor on T cells and the B cell receptor (surface antibody) on B cells recognize different forms of antigen. T cells recognize only small peptides derived from a protein antigen by digestion. B cells generally recognize antigen motifs caused by the tertiary folding of whole soluble protein.

Each part of the antigen that is recognized by either an antibody or a T cell receptor is known as an epitope. Depending on the size of the protein or polysaccharide, there may be hundreds of B cell epitopes (recognized by different antibodies) or T cell epitopes (presented by antigen presenting cells to different T cells) in the same molecule. This actually helps the body have a better response to the antigen as many T and B cells can be activated to respond to one antigen (figure 6).

The antigen fragments are presented on the surface of the cell by a specialized group of molecules. These are encoded in a set of genes known as the major histocompatibility complex (MHC). In humans the same proteins are often referred to as human leukocyte antigens or HLA. MHC is a more specific term as there are lots of antigens on human leukocytes and not all of them are MHC antigens. [10]

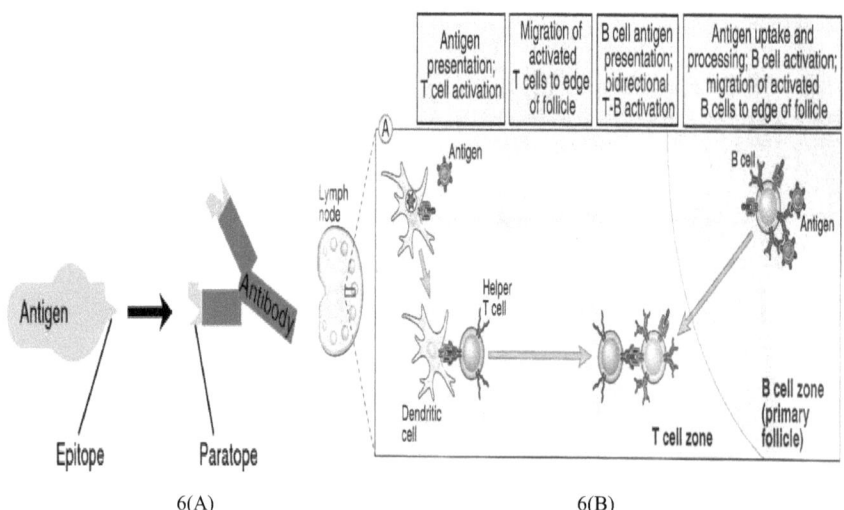

6(A)   6(B)

FIGURE 6: (A) ANTIGEN & ANTIBODY. (From: Copstead and Banasik, 2000.)
(B) RESPONSE OF T & B CELLS TO ANTIGEN (www.biosiva.50webs.org/plasmacell.htm)

[20]

MHC-CLASS I

All cells in the body except red blood cells have MHC class I protein on the surface. Everyone has MHC class I proteins but only identical twins will have identical MHC class I. The genes for the MHC proteins show considerable diversity between people. Class I MHC is a complex of the Class I protein and another protein called ☐2 microglobulin. Since everyone has a different MHC, this allows our body to tell what cells belong to it and what cells are foreign. The function of MHC-I is to sample the internal contents of the cell and show them to the immune system.[10]

MHC-CLASS II

Class II MHC is a complex of proteins only expressed by antigen presenting cells (APC). The function of these proteins is to present an antigen to T helper cells to activate an immune response which will provide both humoral (antibody) and cell mediated immunity. The class II MHC consists of an alpha and a beta chain with a transmembrane segment to hold them on the surface of the cell. At the end farthest from the cell is a cleft where the processed antigen sits. The processed antigen consists of a small peptide of about 13-16 amino acids. MHC-II picks up the antigen that has been ingested (phagocytosed) by the APC[10] (figure 7).

ANTIBODIES:

Antibodies, also called "immunoglobulins", are one of two important protein molecules of the immune system that engage in the recognition of pathogens or other foreign material. This process is called "antigen recognition" and is a pivotal process in the immune response. The other antigen recognition molecule is found on the T cell and is called the T cell receptor (TcR). Antibodies specifically bind to pathogens to bring them to the attention of other parts of the immune system (Complement and phagocytic cells). B cells are the only cells that make antibodies. Antibodies act as recognition units on the surface of B cells (where they are called the B cell receptor) but usually, antibodies are the antigen specific soluble proteins secreted into the blood and tissue by antibody producing cells. Soluble or secreted antibody is structurally slightly different from the antibody on the surface of B cells but the antigen recognition sites are the same.

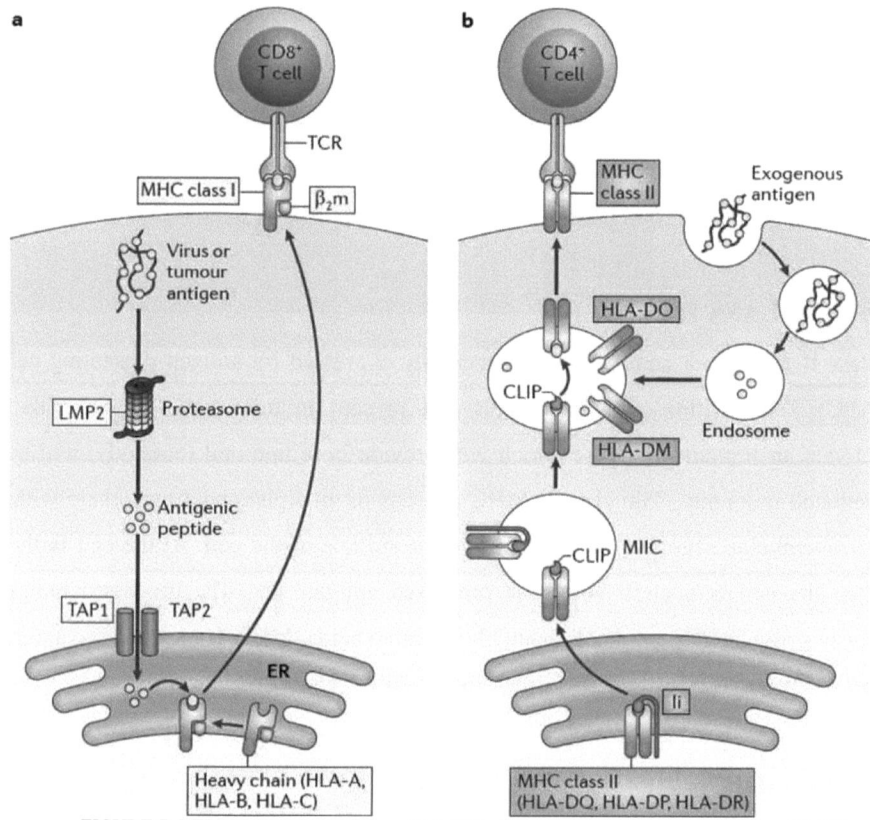

FIGURE 7: MHC PATHWAYS (From: Koichi S. et al., Nature Reviews Immunology 12, 813-820, December 2012)

IgD, IgA, IgM, IgE and IgG – these are the five classes (isotypes) of immunoglobulins. Antibodies recognize antigen.

All antibodies have the same basic Y-shaped structure, with two regions (variable regions) at the tips of the Y that bind to antigen. The stem of the Y is referred to as the constant region and is not involved in antigen binding. The two variable regions contain identical antigen binding sites that, in general, are specific for only one type of antigen. The amino acid sequences of the variable regions of different antibodies, however, are extremely variable. The antibody molecules in the body therefore provide an extremely large repertoire of antigen-binding sites. Each antibody binds to an epitope, which is a restricted part of the antigen. A particular antigen can have several different epitopes or repeated epitopes. Antibodies are specific for the epitopes rather than the whole antigen molecule. The constant region of the antibody (the Fc region) can bind to Fc receptors on phagocytes, so acting as an adapter between the phagocyte and the pathogen. Consequently, if antibody binds to a pathogen, it can link to a phagocyte and promote phagocytosis. The process in which specific binding of an antibody activates an innate immune defence (phagocytosis) is an important example of collaboration between the innate and adaptive immune responses. [11]

Antigen recognition and binding allows antibodies to perform four important effector functions.

1. Opsonisation for phagocytosis
2. Activating Complement
3. Neutralizing toxins
4. Blocking attachment of pathogens to cells or tissue

OPSONIZATION:

This is the process by which bacteria, viruses and small parasites are 'tagged' for destruction by macrophages and neutrophils. Antibodies are the 'tags' (or opsonins) as the antigen binding (Fab) area of the antibody binds to an antigen on the surface of the organism. The other end of the antibody (Fc) binds to receptors on phagocytic cells. The antibody signals the phagocytic cell to engulf and destroy the organism. If the organism is too big to engulf (like a parasitic worm for example) the phagocytic cells will release destructive enzymes and other factors onto the surface of the organism (sometimes called "frustrated phagocytosis). IgG is the most important antibody for this because it is very abundant and fits nicely into the Fc receptor on the surface of the phagocytic cells. IgM and IgA are very poor at this because they are secreted as multimers.

ACTIVATING COMPLEMENT:

It is the process by which antibody binds to an antigen on the surface of a pathogen by its Fab section. The Fc section which is left free, binds to the first component of Complement (C1). This binding of C1 (often called "fixing Complement") activates an enzyme cascade which results in lysis of the organism by the membrane attack complex (the MAC attack). IgM and IgG are very good at activating complement.

NEUTRALIZATION OF TOXINS:

Some pathogens secrete dangerous toxins (such as tetanus toxin). In the circulation, tissues and secretions (such as mucus), antibody will bind to these toxins and neutralize their activity. Antibodies also form easily recognized antibody-toxin complexes which are removed from the body by phagocytosis.

BLOCKING ATTACHMENT:

Antibodies can immobilize and agglutinate infectious agents by binding to their surface antigens and preventing them from attaching to tissues like the intestinal mucosa or from penetrating cells (in the case of viruses).

RECOGNITION OF ANTIGEN:
CLONAL SELECTION:

B and T cells have receptors on their cell surfaces that recognize and bind to specific antigens. When a particular antigen enters the body, it must, by chance, encounter the specific lymphocyte with the appropriate receptor in order to provoke an immune response. The first time a pathogen invades the body; there are only a few B or T cells that may have the receptors that can recognize the invader's antigens. Binding of the antigen to its receptor on the lymphocyte surface, however, stimulates cell division and produces a clone (a population of genetically identical cells). This process is known as clonal selection.[11]

In this first encounter, there are only a few cells that can mount an immune response and the response is relatively weak. This is called a primary immune response. If the primary immune response involves B cells, some become plasma cells that secrete antibodies, and some become memory cells. Because a clone of memory cells specific for that antigen develops after the primary response, the immune response to a second infection by the same pathogen is swifter and stronger. The next time the body is invaded by the same pathogen, the immune system is ready. As a result of the first infection, there is now a large clone of lymphocytes that can recognize that pathogen. This more effective response, elicited by subsequent exposures to an antigen, is called a secondary immune response (figure 8).

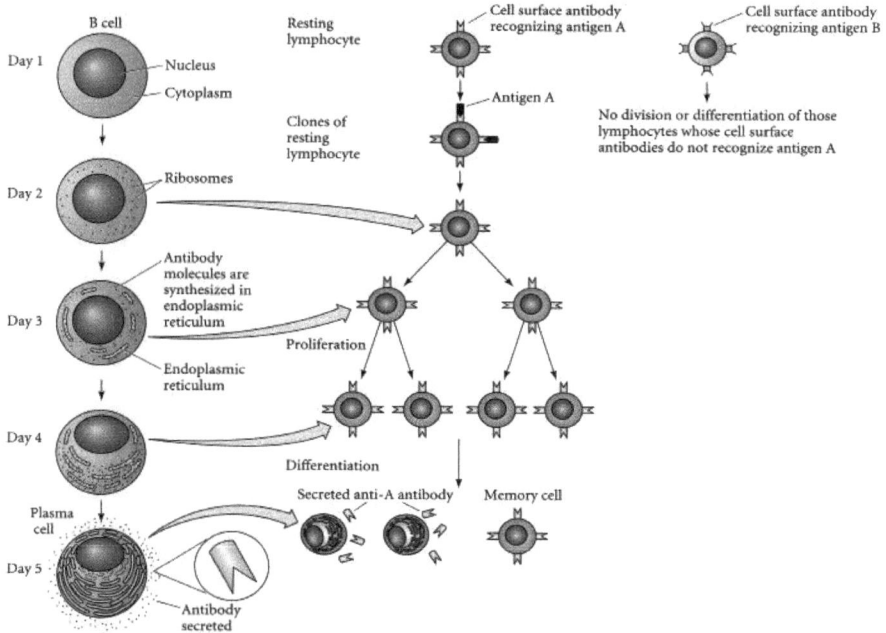

FIGURE 8: CLONAL SELECTION (From: www.helshandidy.wordpress.com/2011/04/28/geniuses-only-artificial-immune-systems-part-ii)

Memory cells can survive for several decades, which is why people rarely contract chicken pox a second time after they have had it once. Memory cells are also the reason that vaccinations are effective. The vaccine triggers the primary response so that if the actual pathogen is encountered later, the large and rapid secondary response occurs and stops the infection before it can start. The viruses causing childhood diseases have surface antigens that change little from year to year, so the same antibody is effective for decades.

IMMUNE EFFECTOR MECHANISM:

There are numerous ways in which the immune system can destroy pathogens, each being suited to a given type of infection at a particular stage of its life cycle. These defence mechanisms are called effector systems which includes:

1. Antibody binding resulting in neutralization.
2. Phagocytosis is promoted by complement and opsonins resulting in ingestion of microbe
3. Cytotoxic reactions are directed against the whole cells that recognized the target cells either by specific antibody bound to the cell surface; or by T cells using their TCRs.

Immune responses to extracellular and intracellular pathogens differ. In dealing with extracellular pathogens, the immune system aims to destroy the pathogen itself and neutralize its products. In dealing with intracellular pathogens, the immune system has two options:

- T cells can destroy the infected cell (i.e. cytotoxicity); or
- T cells can activate the infected cell to deal with the pathogen itself (e.g. helper T cells release cytokines, which activate macrophages to destroy the organisms they have internalized).

Because many pathogens have both intracellular and extracellular phases of infection, different mechanisms are usually effective at different times. For example, the polio virus travels from the gut, through the blood stream to infect nerve cells in the spinal cord. Antibody is particularly effective at blocking the early phase of infection while the virus is in the blood stream, but to clear an established infection CTLs must kill any cell that has become infected[11] (figure 9).

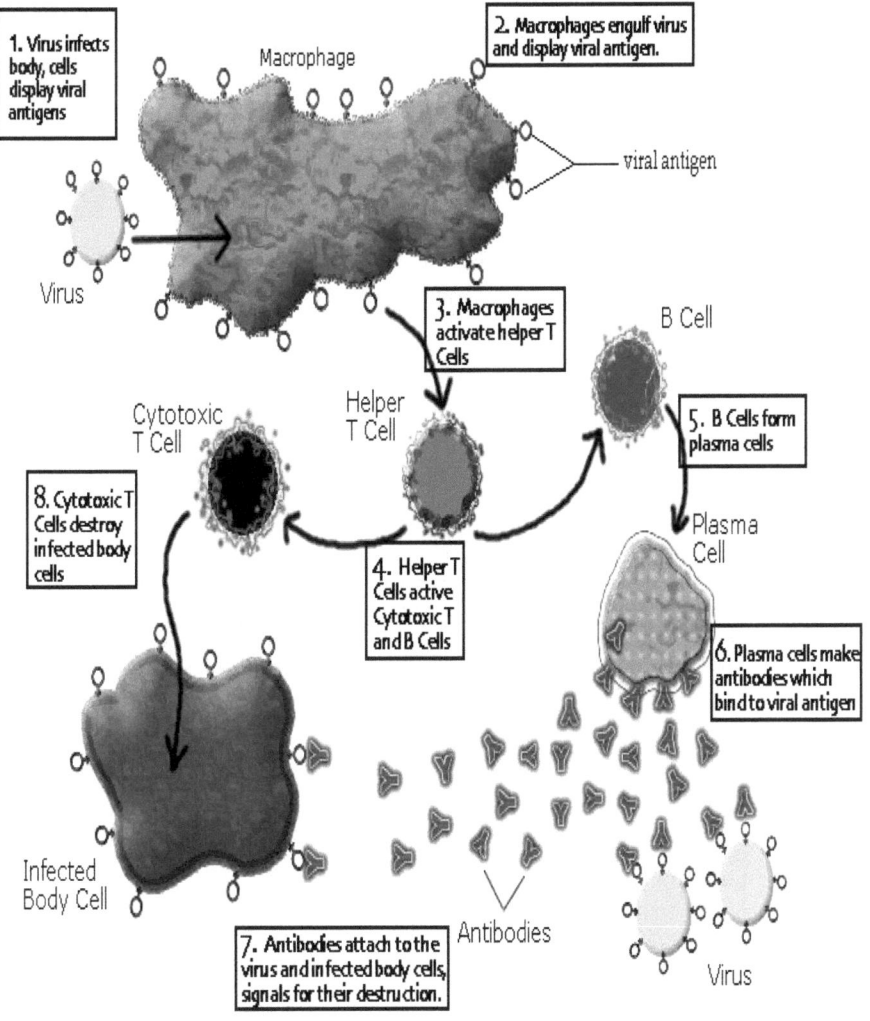

FIGURE 9: THE IMMUNE RESPONSE (From:
www.bcscience8.wikispaces.com/Acquired+Immune+Response)

VACCINATION:

The aim in vaccine development is to alter a pathogen or its toxins in such a way that they become innocuous without losing antigenicity. This is possible because antibodies and T cells recognize particular parts of antigens (the epitopes), and not the whole organism or toxin.

The principle of vaccination is based on two key elements of adaptive immunity, namely specificity and memory (figure 10). Memory cells allow the immune system to mount a much stronger response on second encounter with antigen. This secondary response is both faster to appear and more effective than the primary response. The tetanus bacterium produces a toxin that acts on receptors to cause tetanic contractions of muscle. The toxin can be modified by formalin treatment so that it retains its epitopes, but loses its toxicity. The resulting molecule (known as a toxoid) is used as a vaccine.[11]

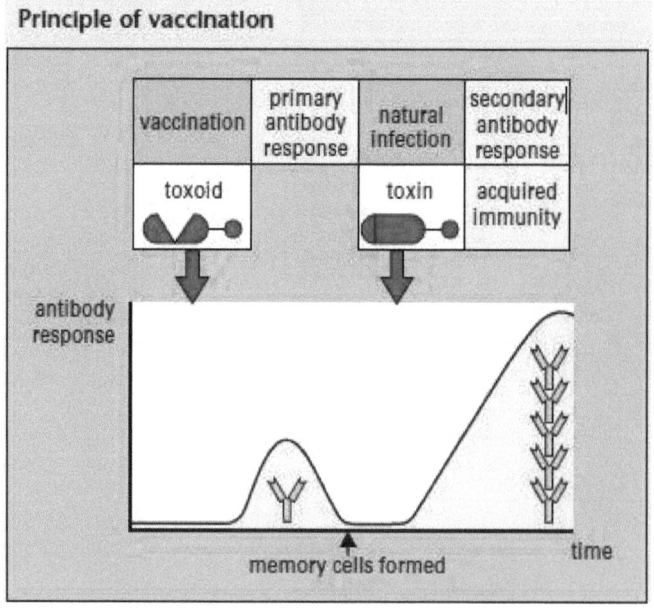

FIGURE 10: VACCINATION PRINCIPLE (From Roitt et al., 2001.)

THE IMMUNE SYSTEM MAY FAIL (IMMUNOPATHOLOGY):

Deficiencies in any part of the system leave the individual exposed to a greater risk of infection, but other parts of the system may partly compensate for such deficiencies. However, there are occasions when the immune system is itself a cause of disease or other undesirable consequences. In essence the immune system can fail in one of three ways, resulting in autoimmunity, immunodeficiency, or hypersensitivity[11] (figure 11).

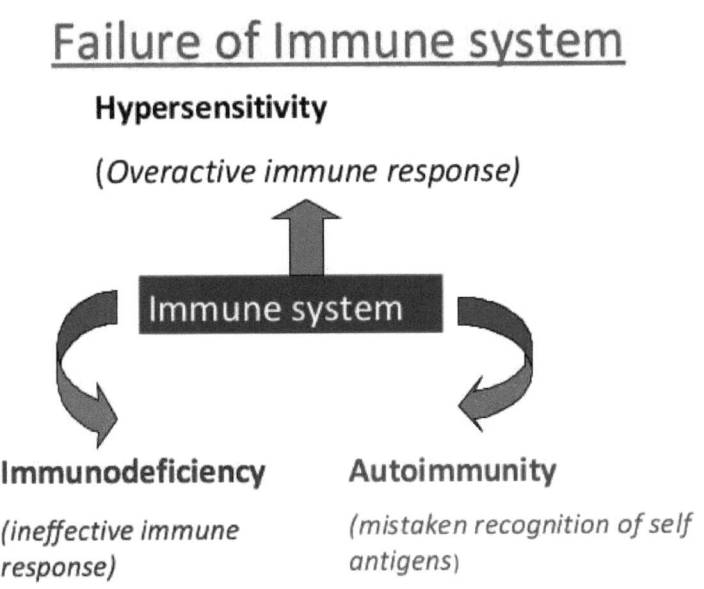

FIGURE 11: FAILURE OF IMMUNE SYSTEM (From: www.slideshare.net/rajukaiti/allergic-conditions)

3. CONCEPTS OF TUMOR IMMUNOLOGY:

The immune system has evolved in order to detect and eliminate pathogens that may do harm to the organism. It serves as a watchdog against transformed cells that may lead to cancer. Interactions between the immune system and malignant cells play an important role in tumorigenesis. Failure of the immune system to detect and reject transformed cells may lead to cancer development. Tumours use multiple mechanisms to escape from immune-mediated rejection. [5]

The immune system has three primary roles in the prevention of tumours.

1. The immune system can protect the host from virus-induced tumours by eliminating or suppressing viral infections.
2. Timely elimination of pathogens and prompt resolution of inflammation can prevent the establishment of an inflammatory environment conducive to tumorigenesis.
3. The immune system can specifically identify and eliminate tumbrels on the basis of their expression of tumour-specific antigens or molecules induced by cellular stress. This third process is referred to as Tumour immunosurveillance. [12]

Immune system is involved in tumour recognition and progression in multiple ways. However, two different models for the immune response to tumours have been proposed:

- The Concept of Immunosurveillance and
- The Danger Model.

Tumour Immunosurveillance is defined as the mechanism in which the immune system identifies cancerous/or precancerous cells and eliminates them before they can cause harm. [12]

According to the immunosurveillance hypothesis, tumours expressing antigens are regarded as "nonself" by the immune system, and a major function of the immune system is to survey the body for the development of malignancy and to eliminate tumour cells as they arise.[5]The self–non-self theory has dominated immunology for 60 years. According to the self–non-self theory, an immune response is triggered against all foreign ("nonself") entities, whereas no immune response is triggered against the organism's own constituents ("self"). [13]

More recently, Polly Matzinger suggested a rival theory, called the "danger theory" or "The Danger Mode theory". Against the self–non-self theory, the danger theory claims that self constituents can trigger an immune response, if they are dangerous (e.g., cellular stress, some autografts, etc.); and non-self constituents can be tolerated, if they are not dangerous (e.g., the foetus or commensal bacteria). This theory claims that immune responses are triggered by "danger signals," or "alarm signals," released by the body's own cells. According to the danger theory every immune response is not due to the presence of "nonself" (i.e., genetically foreign entities), but to the emission, within the organism, of "danger signals."[13]

IMMUNOSURVEILLANCE:

Ehrlich in 1909 first proposed the idea that nascent transformed cells arise continuously in our bodies and that the immune system scans for and eradicates these transformed cells before they are manifested clinically, immune surveillance has been a controversial topic in tumour immunology. In the mid-20th century, experimental evidence that tumours could be repressed by the immune system came from tumour transplantation models. The findings from these models strongly suggested the existence of tumour-associated antigens and formed the basis of immune surveillance, which was postulated by Burnet and Thomas.[14]

After that the functional role of antigen-presenting cells in cross-priming for T-cell activation was demonstrated, and the cancer immune surveillance model was developed. However, the idea of cancer immune surveillance resisted widespread acceptance until the 1990s when experimental animal models using knockout mice validated the existence of cancer immune surveillance in both chemically induced and spontaneous tumours.[14]

Fifty years later as immunologists gained an enhanced understanding of transplantation and tumour immunobiology and immunogenetics, F. Macfarlane Burnet and Lewis Thomas revisited the topic of natural immune protection against cancer. Burnet's thinking was shaped by a consideration of immune tolerance; he believed that tumour cell-specific neo-antigens could provoke an effective immunologic reaction that would eliminate developing cancers. Alternatively, Thomas's early view was evolutionary in nature; he theorized that complex long-lived organisms must possess mechanisms to protect against neoplastic disease similar to those mediating homograft rejections.

Several studies in the 1990s, fuelled by technologic advances in mouse genetics and monoclonal antibody (mAb) production reinvigorated and ultimately validated the cancer immunosurveillance concept and expanded it to incorporate the contributions of both innate and adaptive immunity.

However, there has been a growing recognition that immunosurveillance represents only one dimension of the complex relationship between the immune system and cancer. Recent work has shown that the immune system may also promote the emergence of primary tumours with reduced immunogenicity that is capable of escaping immune recognition and destruction. These findings prompted the development of the cancer immune-editing hypothesis to more broadly encompass the potential host-protective and tumour-sculpting functions of the immune system throughout tumour development. [4]

[32]

Cancer immune surveillance is considered to be an important host protection process to inhibit carcinogenesis and to maintain cellular homeostasis.[14] In spite of tumour immune surveillance, tumours do develop in the presence of a functioning immune system, and therefore the updated concept of tumour immuno-editing is a more complete explanation for the role of the immune system in tumour development.[4]

The cancer immunoediting hypothesis predicts that, whereas one outcome is complete elimination of a developing tumour, another is the generation of a sculpted tumour cell repertoire that displays either reduced immunogenicity or an increased capacity to inhibit protective anti-tumour immune responses.[15]

Cancer immunoediting is a dynamic process composed of three phases:

- Elimination
- Equilibrium and
- Escape.

Elimination represents the classical concept of cancer immunosurveillance, equilibrium is the period of immune-mediated latency after incomplete tumour destruction in the elimination phase, and escape refers to the final outgrowth of tumours that have outstripped immunological restraints of the equilibrium phase[4] (Figure 12-A & 12-B).

ELIMINATION:

Elimination is the hallmark of the original concept in cancer immune surveillance for the successful eradication of developing tumour cells, working in concert with the intrinsic tumour suppressor mechanisms of the nonimmunogenic surveillance process.

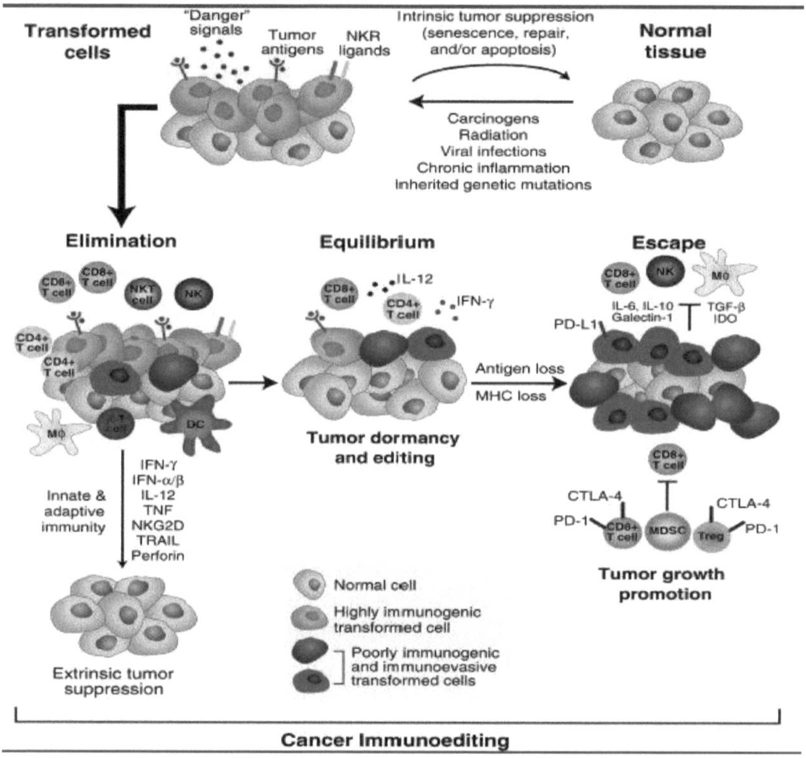

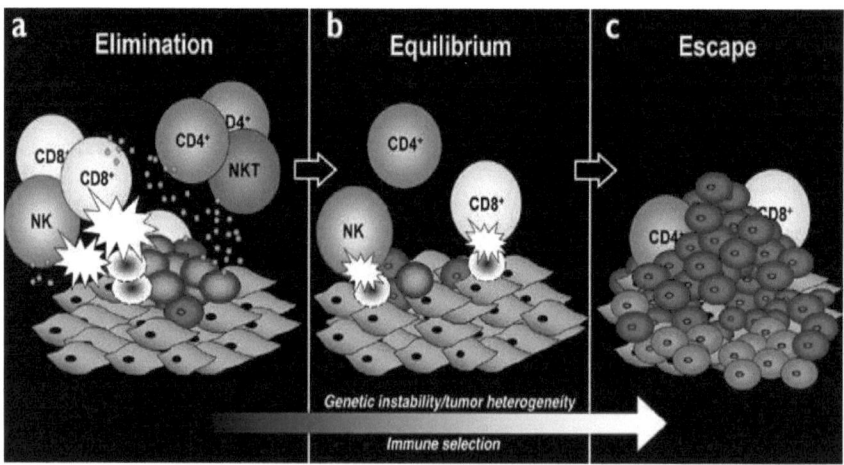

FIGURE 12 (A): CANCER IMMUNOEDITING (From: www.intranet.tdmu.edu.ua)

FIGURE 12 (B): CANCER IMMUNOEDITING (From Dunn et al., Nature Immunology 3,991-998, 2002)

MECHANISM OF CELLS INVOLVED IN ELIMINATION:

Growing tumour Cells, Macrophages & Stromal Cells surrounding the tumour cells

⬇

Release of Inflammatory Cytokines

⬇

Activation of Effector cells such as Natural Killer (NK) cells, T-lymphocytes

⬇

Release of Cytokines by Effector Cells

⬇

Recruitment of more immune cells

⬇

Production of Interleukin-12 (IL-12) & Interferon-c (IFN-c)

⬇

Perforin, FasL- and TRAIL-mediated killing of tumour cells by NK cells

⬇

Release of Tumour Antigens (TAs)

⬇

Leads to Adaptive immune responses

⬇

Maturation of Dendritic Cells & migration to tumour draining lymph nodes

⬇

Enhancement of Antigen presentation to naive T cells

⬇

Clonal expansion of Cytotoxic T lymphocytes (CTLs)

The elimination phase represents the original concept of cancer immunosurveillance. If this phase successfully eradicates the developing tumour, it represents the complete immunoediting process without progression to the subsequent phases. The immunologic rejection of a developing tumour requires an integrated response involving both the innate and adaptive arms of the immune system.

Four phases have been proposed for the elimination process:

First phase:
1. Activation of innate immunity
2. Stromal remodelling – angiogenesis and tissue invasive growth
3. Production of Interferon-c (IFN-c)

Presence of growing tumour & stromal remodelling due to angiogenesis and tissue-invasive growth

Activation of innate immune system

Release of proinflammatory molecules by stromal remodelling and release of chemokines by tumour cells

Summon the Natural Killer (NK) cells, γ δ T cells, NKT cells

γ δ T cells, NKT cells & Macrophages   TCR interaction with NKG2D ligands

or glycolipid-CD1 complexes

Recognition of tumour antigens

Production of Interferon- γ (IFN- γ)

Second Phase:

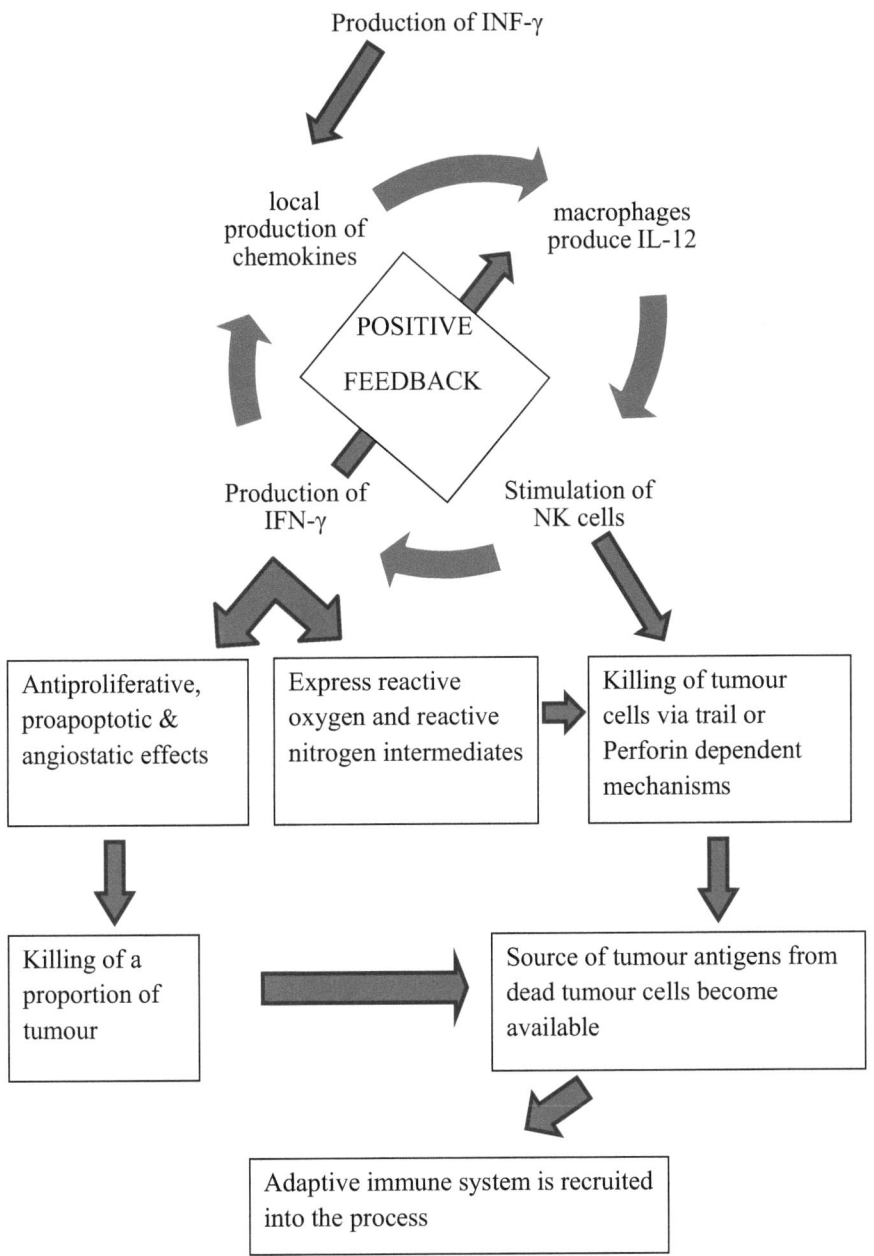

Third Phase:

Tumour antigens liberated by effects of innate immunity

Development of Adaptive immune response

Recruitment of Immature Dendritic Cells (DCs)

Exposure to cytokine milieu

created by innate immunity attack

Interaction with tumour

infiltrating NK cells

Activated DCs acquire tumour antigens by

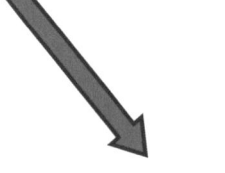

Ingestion of tumour cell debris

proteins.

Indirect mechanisms involving

transfer of tumour cell-derived

heat shock protein or tumour

antigen complexes to DCs

Antigen bearing activated DCs migrate to draining lymph nodes

Induce activation of naive tumour-specific Th1 CD4+ T cells

Th1 facilitate development of tumour-specific CD8+ CTL induced via cross-presentation of antigen tumour peptides on DC MHC class I molecules

[38]

Fourth Phase:

Tumour-specific adaptive immunity
⬇
Provides the host with capacity to completely eliminate the developing tumour

Tumour-specific CD4+ cells
⬇
Produce IL-2, together with host cell IL-15
⬇
Maintain function & viability of tumour-specific CD8+ cells

CD8+ recognize tumour target cells
⬇
Induce tumour cell death by direct and indirect mechanisms
⬇
CD8+ produces INF-γ
⬇
Cell cycle inhibition, apoptosis, angiostasis & induction of macrophage tumoricidal activity

EQUILIBRIUM:

The interactions between the immune system and tumour cells could lead to a variety of outcomes. One outcome is complete elimination of a developing tumour and another is the generation of a sculpted tumour cell repertoire that displays either reduced immunogenicity or an increased capacity to inhibit protective anti-tumour immune responses. This mechanism is called as immunoediting.

During the progression of cancer immunoediting, a stage of equilibrium is attained in which a continuous sculpting of tumour cells produces cells resistant to immune

[39]

effector cells. This process leads to the immune selection of tumour cells with reduced immunogenicity and therefore these cells are more capable of surviving in an immunocompetent host also.

Although random gene mutations may occur within tumours that produce more unstable tumours, these tumour cell variants are less immunogenic, and the immune selection pressure also favours the growth of tumour cell clones with a non-immunogenic phenotype.[14] Equilibrium is probably the longest of the three phases and may occur over a period of many years in humans.[4]

Experiments show that the original tumour cells induced in normal mice and selected by a T-cell-mediated selection process have been adapted to grow in a host with a functional T-cell system, which has eliminated highly immunogenic tumour cells, leaving non-immunogenic tumour cells to grow.[14] The mutator phenotype of tumour cells may result from the three types of genetic instability observed I cancer: nucleotide-excision repair instability (NIN), microsatellite instability (MIN), and chromosome instability (CIN). This genomic instability has the potential to spawn tumour variants of reduced immunogenicity, and some of these will display an enhanced capacity to grow in an unfettered immune selecting environment.[4]

Furthermore, two important issues can be suggested. One is that Perforin-mediated cytotoxicity in T cells contributes more to the elimination of lymphoma cells than epithelial tumour cells, whereas IFN-c-mediated cytotoxicity is directed more to the elimination of mesenchymal tumour cells such as sarcomas. The other is the higher immunogenicity of the tumours derived from immunodeficient mice than those from immnuocompetent mice indicated less immune selection pressure in the tumours derived from immunodeficient mice than in those of immunocompetent mice. Thus, T-cell-mediated elimination has adapted to highly immunogenic tumours, such as chemically and virally induced tumours. On the other hand, the immune selection pressure induces less immunogenic tumour variants that survive and grow in the tumour microenvironment.

Since the equilibrium phase involves the continuous elimination of tumour cells and the production of resistant tumour variants by immune selection pressure, it is likely that equilibrium is the longest of the three processes in cancer immunoediting. In this process, lymphocytes and IFN-c play a critical role in exerting immune selection pressure on tumour cells. During this period of Darwinian selection, many tumour variants from the original are killed but new variants emerge carrying different mutations that increase resistance to immune attack. Since the equilibrium model persists for a long time in the interaction between cancer cells and the host, the transmission of cancer during organ transplantation can be considered.

IMMUNESURVEILLANCE IN HUMANS:

Analysis of individuals with congenital or acquired immunodeficiencies or patients undergoing immunosuppressive therapy has documented a highly elevated incidence of virally induced malignancies such as Kaposi's sarcoma, non-Hodgkin's lymphoma, and cancers of the anal and urogenital tracts compared with immunocompetent individuals.

The study of the incidence of cancers of nonviral origins that may take many years to develop is confounded by the variety of viral and bacterial infections to which these immunodeficient/ immunosuppressed patients are susceptible and by the more rapid appearance of virally induced tumours.

Three lines of evidence to suggest that cancer immunosurveillance indeed occurs in humans:

- Immunosuppressed transplant recipients display higher incidences of nonviral cancers than age-matched immunocompetent control populations;
- Cancer patients can develop spontaneous adaptive and innate immune responses to the tumours that they bear, and

[41]

- The presence of lymphocytes within the tumour can be a positive prognostic indicator of patient survival.

DANGER THEORY:

To assess the validity of the danger theory, it seems essential to define precisely what a "danger". Matzinger and her colleagues use several terms, which they apparently interpret as equivalent: "danger," "damage," "stress," "injury," "necrosis," "inappropriate (/non- physiological/bad) cell death," etc.

Matzinger and colleagues' theory is much more precise if its central claim is that every immune response is due to *damages* to the organism's cells or tissues. Indeed, it is easier to define what a "damage" is (for an organism, a tissue or a cell) than what a "danger" is. In fact, this is the interpretation that Matzinger proposes when she describes the molecular details of her theory. As Matzinger suggests, the claim that immune responses were due to "danger" was merely a theoretical suggestion, while the idea that they are due to "damages" has led to several experimental investigations. Therefore, in order to assess the "danger theory," the main concern is to define "damage" signals. [16]

As a hypothesis of danger theory, it was considered that cellular transformation did not provide sufficient proinflammatory signals to activate the immune system in response to a developing tumour. In the absence of such signals, there is often no immune response and tolerance may develop. However, recent studies indicate that danger signals such as uric acid, the potential toll-like receptor ligands such as heat-shock proteins or a ligand transfer molecule in the signalling cascade induced by CpG DNA, and extracellular matrix (ECM) derivatives, may induce pro-inflammatory responses that activate innate immune responses to foreign pathogens.

Danger signals are thought to act by stimulating the maturation of DCs so that they can present foreign antigens and stimulate T lymphocytes. Dying mammalian cells have also been found to release danger signals of unknown identity. Of note, although local limited inflammation may be involved in initiating immune responses, excessive inflammation may promote tumour progression in steady-state conditions. This may be in part because of the anti-inflammatory reactions in antigen-presenting cells, which release anti-inflammatory cytokines such as IL-10 and transforming growth factor-b (TGF-b) that inhibits the activation of effector cells.[17]

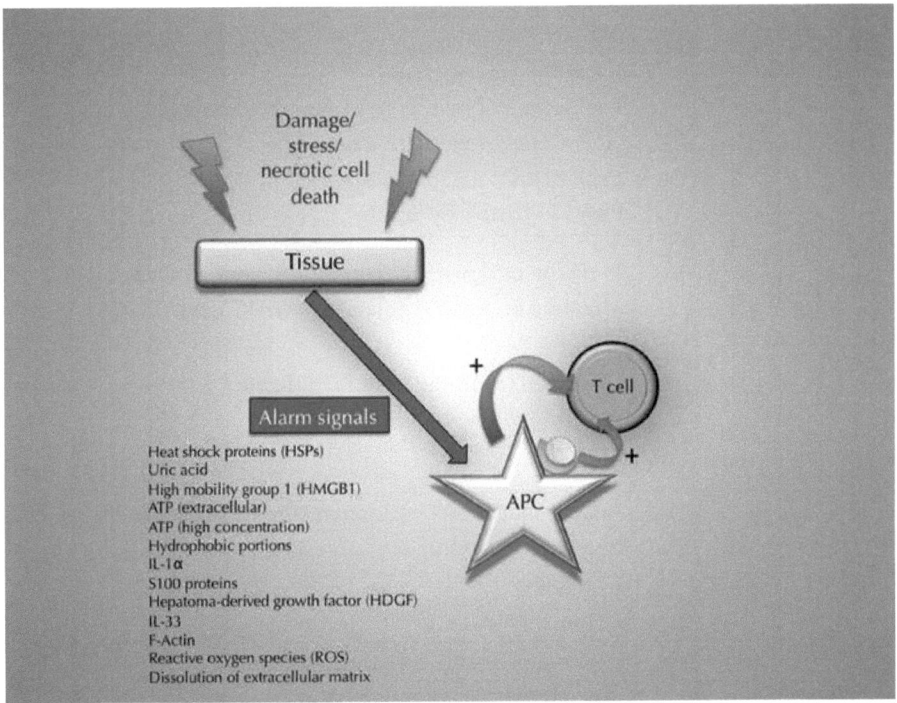

FIGURE 13: THE PRINCIPLE OF THE TRIGGERING OF AN IMMUNE RESPONSE ACCORDING TO THE DANGER (OR "DAMAGE") THEORY. (From: Pradeu T and Cooper EL (2012), The danger theory: 20 years later. *Front. Immun.* 3:287)

4. ESCAPE OF TUMOURS:

Edited tumour cells surviving the equilibrium phase of the cancer immunoediting process enter the escape phase where tumour growth proceeds unrestrained by immune pressure.[4]Interactions between the immune system and malignant cells play an important role in tumorigenesis. Failure of the immune system to detect and reject transformed cells may lead to cancer development. Tumours use multiple mechanisms to escape from immune-mediated rejection. Multiple mechanisms have been identified that tumours use to escape from rejection.[5]

STRATEGY	MECHANISM
IGNORANCE	Lack of danger signals Lack of tumour antigens in lymphoid organs Growth in immune privileged sites Lack of adhesion molecules Physical barrier by stroma
IMPAIRED ANTIGEN PRESENTATION	Mutation or down regulation of tumour antigens Mutation or down regulation of MHC genes
EXPRESSION OF IMMUNOSUPPRESSIVE FACTORS & MOLECULES	Cytokines (TGF-ß, IL-10, VEGF, etc.) Prostaglandins RCASI
TOLERANCE INDUCTION	Angery induction (Lack of co stimulatory molecules) Immune deviation Regulatory T cells T cell deletion
APOPTOSIS RESISTANCE	Expression of anti-apoptotic molecules Down regulation & mutation of pro-apoptotic molecules CD95L expression
COUNTERATTACK	Expression of other death-receptor ligands

(Figure 14)

Escape: immune system sculpts tumors

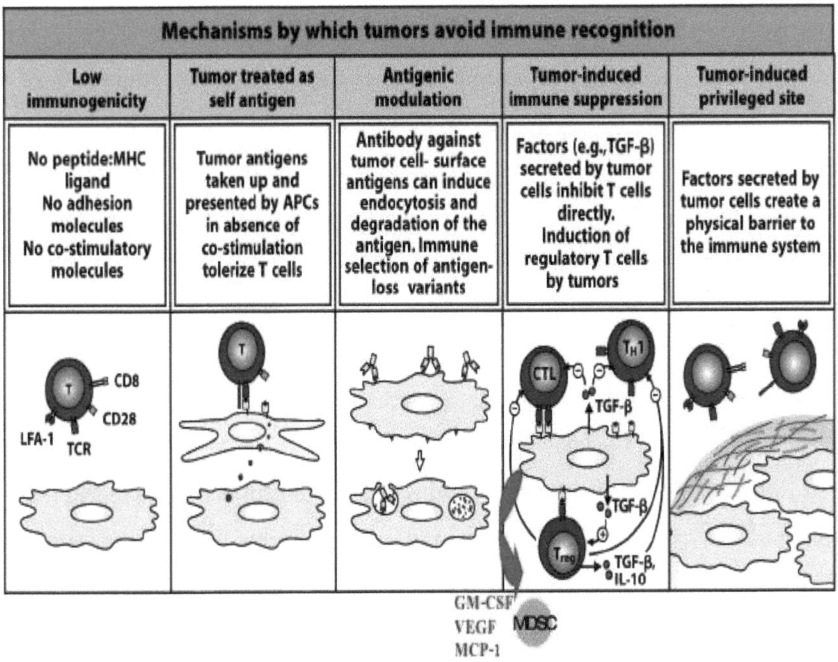

Mechanisms by which tumors avoid immune recognition				
Low immunogenicity	**Tumor treated as self antigen**	**Antigenic modulation**	**Tumor-induced immune suppression**	**Tumor-induced privileged site**
No peptide:MHC ligand No adhesion molecules No co-stimulatory molecules	Tumor antigens taken up and presented by APCs in absence of co-stimulation tolerize T cells	Antibody against tumor cell- surface antigens can induce endocytosis and degradation of the antigen. Immune selection of antigen-loss variants	Factors (e.g.,TGF-β) secreted by tumor cells inhibit T cells directly. Induction of regulatory T cells by tumors	Factors secreted by tumor cells create a physical barrier to the immune system

GM-CSF
VEGF MDSC
MCP-1

FIGURE 14: IMMUNE ESCAPE OF TUMORS (From: Immunology, 7th Edition, Garland Science 2008)

IGNORANCE:

Despite presentation of antigens by malignant cells and the presence of immune cells that could potentially react against these cells, in many cases the immune system does not get activated but "ignores" the tumour. According to the danger model, APC may not get activated in this situation due to of a lack of danger signals. Other factors may also contribute to immunological ignorance. The immune system ignores tumour cells, which fail to migrate to lymph nodes and fail to activate T cells directly. In addition, tumours growing in immune privileged sites such as the brain or the eye are not surveyed by the immune system. Down-regulation of adhesion molecules in

[45]

malignant tissue may inhibit immune infiltration and thus may also contribute to immunological ignorance.[5]

IMPAIRED ANTIGEN PRESENTATION:

One strategy to escape from the adaptive immune response is by impaired antigen presentation. Defects in antigen presentation are more pronounced in metastatic lesions than in the primary tumour. Expression of the tumour antigens is down-regulated, leading to enhanced tumour incidence and metastasis. Mutations of the antigen can result in the escape from the initial response and contribute to the heterogenecity of tumour lesions. This heterogenous expression hinders the establishment of an efficient specific immune response. Down-regulation of LMP2 (Low Molecular mass Polypeptide-2) and LMP7 changes the variety of peptides presented by MHC (Major Histocompatibility Complex) molecules.

TAP (transporter associated with antigen processing) and tapasin are the two proteins associated with loading antigen peptides onto MHC-1 molecules. Deficiency of TAP results in loss of MHC-1 expression, resulting in tumour formation. Reduced MHC-1 expression also prevents recognition of tumour cells by the immune system as tumours often have heterogenous pattern of MHC-1 expression. Point mutations, gene rearrangements or deletion and defects in transcriptional regulation lead to loss of an MHC allele or locus. Mutations of ß2 microglobulins subunits can cause total loss of MHC-1 expression which makes the tumour, target site for NK cell attack. Consequently, the tumour needs further mechanisms to resist NK cell-mediated lysis, such as the expression of MHC-1 replacements.[20]

EXPRESSION OF IMMUNOSUPPRESSIVE FACTORS:

Immunosuppressive factors are expressed by tumour cells themselves or by noncancerous cells such as immune, epithelial or stromal cells and most prominent of these factors is transforming growth factor ß (TGF- ß). TGF- ß affects proliferation, activation & differentiation of cells of innate and adaptive immunity and inhibits the

[46]

anti-tumour immune response. RCAS1 (Receptor Binding Cancer antigen expressed on SiSo cells) inhibits proliferation and induces apoptosis in T cells, resulting in immune evasion of tumours. Vascular Endothelial Growth Factor (VEGF) inhibits the differentiation of progenitors into dendritic cells. Prostaglandins, interleukin-10 (IL-10), macrophage colony stimulating factor, etc. are immunosuppressive factors released by tumour cells.[21]

TOLERANCE INDUCTION:

In healthy organisms, self-reactive T cells are tolerated mainly by deletion in the thymus, by a process known as Central tolerance. Peripheral tolerance induction is complex multistep process involving four major mechanisms.

First mechanism is the induction of anergy. Activation of T cells requires signals expressed through binding of a peptide-MHC complex to the TCR and binding of co stimulatory molecules (e.g. B7) to their ligands (CD28) on T cell surface. T cell bound to peptide-MHC complex via TCR is rendered anergic and does not become activated without sufficient costimulation. Many tumour cells do not express co stimulatory molecules and thus induce anergy in anti-tumour lymphocytes.

Second mechanism of tolerance induction is immune deviation. The immune response is driven toward a Th2 humoral response pathway away from a Th1 response required for efficient tumour rejection by cytotoxic T cells. This depends on secretion of TGF-ß and IL-10 or on the presentation of tumour antigen by B cells on CD4$^+$ Th cells.

Third mechanism of tolerance induction is T-cell deletion. Repetitive stimulation of T cells with antigens, peptides, superantigens or allogeneic cells or direct restimulation of the TCR by anti-CD3 antibodies has been shown to induce tolerance by T cell deletion. It is mediated via CD95/CD95L death system. This process is referred to as activation-induced cell death (AICD). AICD, as a result of chronic stimulation with the tumour antigen may contribute to immune escape.

Fourth mechanism used by tumours to induce tolerance is related to apoptosis. Malignant cells have changes in the expression of molecules involved in apoptosis signalling, resulting in resistance of the tumour to the killing mechanisms of the immune system. Tumours adopt a killing mechanism from cytotoxic immune cells to delete the attacking anti-tumour lymphocytes, a concept called "tumour counterattack".[22]

RESISTANCE TO APOPTOSIS AND IMMUNE ESCAPE:

In an immune-competent host, tumour cells are selected for resistance against the effector mechanisms of the immune system, a concept known as immunoselection or immunoediting. Although many mechanisms of tumour resistance to apoptosis have been identified, only a few of them have directly been shown to be involved in immune escape. One strategy tumours use to acquire apoptosis resistance is the overexpression of antiapoptotic molecules. FLICE-inhibitory proteins (FLIP) interferes with apoptosis induction at the level of death receptors, but do not prevent apoptosis by Perforin/granzyme. Human melanomas and Epstein-Barr virus positive Burkitt's lymphoma cells express high levels of FLIP. Increased ratio of FLIP to caspase-8 is seen in Burkitt's lymphoma, which is correlated with resistance to CD95-mediated apoptosis. Kaposi Sarcoma associated herpes virus (KSHV) encodes viral FLIPs (v-FLIPs) and KSHV-FLIP promotes tumour establishment and growth in immunocompetent mice by prevention of death receptor-induced apoptosis triggered by T cells.[5]

In cooperation with c-Myc or promyelocytic leukemia retinoic acid receptor α, Bcl-2 contributes to tumorigenesis. High Bcl-2 expression correlates with the grade of malignancy of human tumours. The tumour associated viruses like Epstein-Barr virus

[48]

and human KSHV encode proteins that are homologus of Bcl-2. Both proteins BHRF1 and KSbcl-2, respectively, have an antiapoptotic function and enhance survival of the infected cells.

The IAP family member Survivin is found in the vast majority of human tumours and has an antiapoptotic activity along with an apparent role in cell cycle. Expression of a mutant of Survivin that could not be phosphorylated induces cytochrome c release and cell death. cIAP2, another IAP family member, is affected by translocation t(11;18)(q21;q21) and has a role in oncogenesis of mucosa-associated lymphoid tissue (MALT) lymphoma.

Tumour cells also resist killing by direct interference with the Perforin/granzyme pathway. Serine protease inhibitor PI-9/SPI-6 inhibits granzyme B and overexpressions result in resistance of tumour cells to cytotoxic lymphocytes and to immune escape. Neutralization or impairing of the death-inducing stimuli is another mechanism used by tumours to escape from immune system. Two distinct soluble receptors, soluble CD95 (sCd95) and decoy receptor 3 (DcR3) inhibit CD95 signalling completely. High sCD95 serum levels are associated with poor prognosis in melanoma patients. Binding of Perforin to the tumour cell membrane is impaired and this makes tumour cells completely resistance toward NK cell mediated cytotoxicity.[5]

Tumours can acquire apoptosis resistance by down regulation or inactivation of proapoptotic molecules. Oncogenic Ras and p53 aberrations down-regulates or leads to loss of expression of CD95 gene. Point mutations in cytoplasmic death domain of CD95 and deletion lead to a truncated form of the death receptor. Mutated forms of CD95 interfere in a dominant negative way with apoptosis induction via CD95. In certain tumours, Bax (proapoptotic Bcl-2 family member) is mutated leading to loss of expression and poor response rate to chemotherapy and shorter survival. Bax is relevant primarily for apoptosis stimuli such as chemotherapy or p53 and not for apoptosis triggered by the immune system.

Tumour cells use many mechanisms to acquire apoptosis resistance which is not only relevant for tumorigenesis and resistance to chemotherapy, but also influences immunosurveillance and immunotherapy.[5]

TUMOR COUNTERATTACK:

Tumour cells may not only resist destruction by the immune system passively, but may also kill tumour-infiltrating lymphocytes actively to suppress the anti-tumour response, a phenomenon called "tumour counterattack". CD95L is the weapon used by tumours to delete CD95 sensitive immune cells. CD95L is expressed in immune-privileged sites, e.g., the eye and the testis. Thus, in the eye a high percentage of human corneal transplants are accepted without tissue matching or immunosuppressive therapy. CD95L is used to render a transplanted tissue an immune privileged site.[5]

Tumour cells expressing only soluble CD95L do not elicit a neutrophilic infiltration whereas tumour cells expressing a noncleavable membrane bound form of CD95L are rapidly rejected. CD95L acts on surrounding cells to induce the production of granulocyte chemoattractants. CD95L induces the processing and release of IL-1ß, which is responsible for the infiltration by neutrophils. CD95L also acts on resident macrophages, leading to increased production of IL-1ß and macrophage inflammatory proteins.

Many studies of tumour counterattack have been published, but the results are contradictory, and therefore do not clarify whether tumour counterattack is a relevant immune escape mechanism. Additional factors may influence the outcome of CD95L expression on tumours and thus level and time-point of CD95L expression is particularly relevant. Overexpression of CD95L leads to rejection by neutrophils, whereas physiological levels may not induce neutrophilic infiltration but still is sufficient to delete anti-tumour lymphocytes. Death ligand TRAIL suppresses tumour-specific T cell responses in a similar manner as CD95L. The membrane protein RCAS1 not only inhibits proliferation, but also inhibits apoptosis in T cell.[23]

A macroscopic tumour is heterogenous, and different cells within the tumour may also use different immune escape mechanisms including apoptosis resistance, impaired antigen presentations, secretion of immunosuppressive factors, and other strategies whereas multiple mechanisms may develop in a single tumour cell. Deeper insight into the molecular mechanisms underlying tumour immune escape may finally lead to novel therapeutic approaches that will be used for the benefit of cancer patients.[5]

5. <u>IMMUNOTHERAPY</u>

Immunotherapy is also sometimes called *biologic therapy* or *biotherapy*. It is the treatment that uses certain parts of the immune system to fight diseases such as cancer. This can be done in a couple of ways:

- Stimulating own immune system to work harder or smarter to attack cancer cells
- Giving immune system components, such as man-made immune system proteins.[18]

The study of immunotherapy in cancer spans several decades with hundreds of clinical trials, using many different immuno-stimulatory strategies and modalities for vaccine delivery. Immunotherapy has potential application in the treatment of cancer, where it has been demonstrated to induce both clinical responses and robust immunological responses in sub-groups of treated patients.

The first example of immunotherapy for cancer applied in a clinical setting was credited to William Coley at the end of the 19th century. Coley hypothesised that immunity raised in response to bacterial infection may be an important factor in the rejection of established tumours, an idea that led him to the development of the killed streptococcal preparations which later became known as Coley's Toxins. Using the principles of Coley, bladder cancer is treated with intravesicular Bacillus Calmette Guerin (BCG). The majority of immunotherapy research focuses on the 'vaccine' approach and targets tumour-specific antigens. One of the major breakthroughs in the field was the identification of first tumour antigens in mice and humans that could be specifically recognised by lytic T-cell clones.

The development of strategies to overcome the natural tendency of tumours to vary their antigenic profile and to suppress immune responses is a key issue in the design of immunological therapies for cancer. (Figure 15) It is well established that tumours down-regulate many of the molecules involved in processing and presentation of peptide on major histocompatibility complex (MHC) class I, and that changes occur in the antigenic profile of tumours as they progress and metastasise.[9]

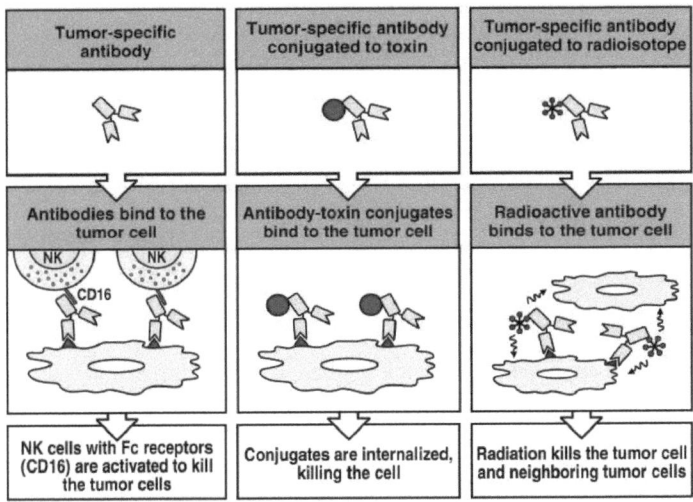

FIGURE 15: IMMUNOTHERAPY (From: www.intranet.tdmu.edu.ua/main principles of prescription of the immune medicine)

Germs such as viruses, bacteria, and parasites have substances on their outer surfaces, such as certain proteins, that are not normally found in the human body. The immune system sees these foreign substances as antigens. Cancer cells are also different from normal cells in the body. They often have unusual substances on their outer surfaces that can act as antigens. But the immune system is much better at recognizing and attacking germs than cancer cells. Germs are very different from normal human cells and are often easily seen as foreign, but cancer cells and normal cells have fewer clear differences. Because of this the immune system may not always recognize cancer cells as foreign. Cancer cells are less like soldiers of an invading army and more like traitors within the ranks of the human cell population.

Clearly the immune system's normal ability to fight cancer is limited, because many people with healthy immune systems still develop cancer. The immune system may not see the cancer cells as foreign because the cancer cells (and their antigens) are not different enough from those of normal cells. Sometimes the immune system recognizes the cancer cells, but the response may not be strong enough to destroy the cancer. Cancer cells themselves may also give off substances that keep the immune system in check.

Cancer treatment methods include surgical therapy, chemotherapy, hormonal therapy, radiation therapy, adjuvant therapy and Immunotherapy. Ancient surgeons knew that cancer would usually come back after it was removed by surgery. During the last decades of the 20th century, surgeons developed new methods for cancer treatment by combining surgery with chemotherapy and/or radiation. Over the years, use of many chemotherapy drugs has resulted in the successful treatment of many types of cancers. Now new approaches are being studied to reduce the side effects of chemotherapy including use of, (a) new combinations of drugs, (b) liposomal and monoclonal antibody therapy to target specifically cancer cells, (c) chemoprotective agents to reduce chemotherapy side effects, (d) hematopoietic stem cell transplantation and (e) agents that overcome multidrug resistance. Adjuvant therapy is the use of chemotherapy after surgery to destroy the few remaining cancer cells in the body.[18]

IMMUNOTHERAPY:

Use of biological agents that mimic some of the natural signals that body uses to control tumour growth is called immunotherapy. These natural biological agents can now be produced in the laboratory including interferons, interleukins, cytokines, endogenous angioinhibitors and antigens. There are many types of cancer treatments that could be thought of as immunotherapy. The main types of immunotherapy being used to treat cancer are:

- **Monoclonal antibodies:** These are man-made versions of immune system proteins. Antibodies can be very useful in treating cancer because they can be designed to attack a very specific part of a cancer cell.
- **Cancer vaccines:** Vaccines are substances put into the body to start an immune response against certain diseases. They are usually thought as being given to .healthy people to help prevent infections. But some vaccines may help prevent or treat cancer.
- **Non-specific immunotherapies:** These treatments boost the immune system in a very general way, but this may still result in more activity against cancer cells.

Monoclonal antibodies

One way the immune system normally attacks foreign substances in the body is by making large numbers of different antibodies. Many copies of a specific antibody can be made in the laboratories which are known as *monoclonal antibodies* (mAbs or moAbs). These antibodies can be useful in fighting diseases because they can be designed specifically to only target a certain antigen, such as one that is found on cancer cells.

A major advantage of these drugs is that because they are so specific, they may have only mild side effects, unlike some other cancer treatments. Identification of right antigen is necessary for attack and for cancer this is not always easy, and so far mAbs have proven to be more useful against some cancers than others.

Two types of monoclonal antibodies are used in cancer treatments:

- *Naked mAbs* are antibodies that work by themselves. There is no drug or radioactive material attached to them. These are the most commonly used mAbs at this time. E.g. Alemtuzumab (Campath) is an antibody that binds to the CD52 antigen, which is found on immune cells called B cells and T cells and is used to treat some patients with chronic lymphocytic leukemia.

- *Conjugated mAbs* are those joined to a chemotherapy drug, radioactive particle, or a toxin (a substance that poisons cells). These mAbs work, at least in part, by acting as homing devices to take these substances directly to the cancer cells. The mAb circulates in the body until it can find and hook onto the target antigen. It then delivers the toxic substance where it is needed most. This lessens the damage to normal cells in other parts of the body. Conjugated mAbs are also sometimes referred to as *tagged*, *labelled*, or *loaded* antibodies. They can be divided into groups as follows.

⇒ mAbs with radioactive particles attached are referred to as *radiolabeled*, and treatment with this type of antibody is known as *radioimmunotherapy* (RIT). E.g. Ibritumomab tiuxetan (Zevalin) and tositumomab (Bexxar) are antibodies against the CD20 antigen with different radioactive particle attached and can be used to treat some types of non-Hodgkin lymphoma.

⇒ mAbs with chemotherapy drugs attached are referred to as *chemolabeled*. E.g. Brentuximab vedotin (Adcetris), approved by FDA, targets the CD30 antigen and is used to treat Hodgkin lymphoma and anaplastic large cell lymphoma that is no longer responding to other treatments.

⇒ mAbs attached to cell toxins are called *immunotoxins*. E.g. denileukin diftitox (Ontak) consists of an immune system protein known as interleukin-2 (IL-2) attached to a toxin from the germ that causes diphtheria and is used to treat lymphoma of the skin.

Monoclonal antibodies are given intravenously (injected into a vein). Compared with the side effects of chemotherapy, the side effects of naked mAbs are usually fairly mild and are often more like an allergic reaction. Fever, chills, weakness, headache, nausea, vomiting, diarrhoea, low blood pressure, rashes are possible side effects of monoclonal antibodies. Conjugated antibodies may pack more of a punch than naked mAbs, but they often cause more side effects. The side effects depend on which type of substance they're attached to.[18]

CANCER VACCINES:

Cancer vaccines work the same way as the vaccines given to healthy people to help prevent infections, such as measles and mumps. Some strains of the human papilloma virus (HPV) have been linked to cervical, anal, throat, and some other cancers. Vaccines against HPV may help protect against some of these cancers. These types of vaccines are only useful for cancers known to be caused by infections. A cancer treatment vaccine uses cancer cells, parts of cells, or pure antigens to increase the immune response against cancer cells that are already in the body. Vaccines are often combined with other substances or cells called *adjuvants* that help boost the immune response even further. Cancer vaccines don't just boost the immune system in general; they cause the immune system to attack cells with one or more specific antigens.

Most tumour cell vaccines are *autologous*, meaning the vaccine is made from killed tumour cells taken from the same person in whom they will later be used. In other words, cells are taken during surgery, the vaccine is made from them in a lab, and the cells are injected back into the patient. Some vaccines are *allogeneic*, meaning the cells for the vaccine come from someone other than the patient being treated. Allogeneic vaccines are easier to make than autologous vaccines. Antigen vaccines may be specific for a certain type of cancer, but they are not made for a specific patient like autologous cell vaccines are. Scientists often combine several antigens in a vaccine to try to get a stronger immune response.

[57]

Dendritic cell vaccines are autologous vaccines (made from the person in whom they will be used), and must be made individually for each patient. The process used to create them is complex and expensive. Doctors remove some immune cells from the blood and expose them in the lab to cancer cells or cancer antigens, as well as to other chemicals that turn them into dendritic cells and help them grow. The dendritic cells are then injected back into the patient, where they should provoke an immune response to cancer cells in the body.[18]

Vector-based vaccines use special delivery systems (called *vectors*) to make them more effective. Vectors are helpful in making vaccines for a number of reasons. First, they may be used to deliver more than one cancer antigen at a time, which may make the body's immune system more likely to mount a response. Second, vectors such as viruses and bacteria may trigger their own immune responses from the body, which may help make the overall immune response even stronger. Finally, these vaccines may be easier and less expensive to make than some other vaccines.

Non-specific immunotherapies and adjuvants:

Non-specific immunotherapies do not target a certain cell or antigen. They stimulate the immune system in a very general way, but this may still result in more activity against cancer cells. E.g. The FDA has approved IFN-α for use against Kaposi sarcoma, Follicular non-hodgkin's lymphoma, hairy cell leukemia etc. Granulocyte Macrophage – Colony Stimulating Factor (GM-CSF) is also being tested against cancer as a non-specific immunotherapy and as an adjuvant given with other types of immunotherapies.

Advantages:
- They can be given alone or as adjuvants to boost the immune system.
- They can be used to lessen the side effects of chemotherapeutic agents.

- They can help the bone marrow to make more leukocytes, Red blood cells or platelets

Targeted Cancer Treatments:

Until late 1990's most of the drugs used in cancer therapy worked by killing cancer cells. Unfortunately chemotherapy agents used, also killed some normal cells and had a greater effect on cancer cells.

Growth signal inhibitors

Abnormal levels of growth factors and changes in growth factors signalling leads to abnormal behaviour of cancer cells. Growth factors will inform cells when to grow and divide. Present targeted therapies that block growth factor signals are trastuzumab, gefitinib, imatinib and cetuximab.

Drugs that induce apoptosis

Apoptosis is a natural process through which cellular DNA gets damaged and cells ultimately will die whereas apoptosis inducing drugs can force cancer cells to die without DNA repair.[18]

Endogenous angioinhibitors

Angiogenesis is the formation of new blood vessels from existing vessel. Normally angiogenesis is a healthy process, that help the body to heal wounds and repair damaged body tissues, whereas in cancerous condition this process supports new blood vessel formation that provide a tumour with its own blood supply, nutrients and allow it to grow. Angioinhibition is a form of targeted therapy that uses drugs to stop tumours from making new blood vessels. This concept was first proposed by Judah Folkman from Harvard Medical School, but it wasn't until 2004 that the first angioinhibitor bevicizumab was approved for clinical use. At present there are about

25 endogenous angioinhibitors in clinical trials and many more in preclinical studies for the treatment of cancer. There are two general categories of angioinhibitors:

(i)   Antibodies or small molecules that target pro-angiogenic factors of tumour cells such as VEGF, bFGF or PDGF, and

(ii) Endogenous angioinhibitors such as thrombopondin-1, angiostatin, interferons, endostatin, arresten, canstatin and tumstatin that inhibit angiogenesis by targeting vascular endothelial cells. We have discovered several angioinhibitors signalling mechanisms and their significance for the treatment of cancer.

Future Cancer Treatments:

The growth in knowledge of cancer biology has led to remarkable progress in cancer early detection, treatment and prevention in recent years. Cancer research is currently advancing on so many fronts that are highlighted below.

Antiangiogenic chemotherapy

Angioinhibitors are being used in combination with conventional chemotherapy. It is very important to know the synergism between angioinhibitors and chemotherapeutic agents used. E.g. it is very important to know whether bisphosphonates are synergistic with certain natural angioinhibitors such as angiostatin, endostatin, thrombospondin, arresten, canstatin tumstatin etc. Foods that have high levels of natural angioinhibitors are also being tested for prevention of cancer.

Nanotechnology

It is the use of extremely tiny particles for diagnostic imaging to know the more accurate location of tumours and for delivering drugs more specifically and effectively into cancer cells.

RNA expression profiling and proteomics

RNA expression profiling permits scientists to determine relative amounts of numerous RNA molecules at one time. Knowing what proteins or RNA molecules are present in cancer cell can help to determine how a cell is behaving and often can help to predict which drugs that particular tumour cell is likely to respond.

Immunotherapy includes a wide variety of treatments that work in different ways. Some seem to work by boosting the body's immune system in a very general way. Others help train the immune system to attack cancer cells specifically. Immunotherapy seems to work better for some types of cancer than for others. It is used by itself to treat some cancers, but for many cancers it seems to work best when used along with other types of treatment.[18]

During the past two decades, the paradigm for cancer treatment has evolved from relatively nonspecific cytotoxic agents to selective, mechanism-based therapeutics. Our knowledge of antitumour immune control has recently progressed rapidly, and a new vision of immunotherapy has emerged from new concepts, medical strategies, medications and medical devices. It is likely that in the coming years the reciprocal movement from bench to bed and from bed to bench will continue to accelerate both the expansion of scientific knowledge and the development of innovative treatments.[19]

Finally winning the war against human cancer has been the focal point of present medical research. Single "cure-all" drug for cancer has not yet been developed, even though many new cancer treatment methods and drug targets have been discovered. More research studies and different clinical trials are the key to find a cure for cancer. The complexity of cancer disease demands scientific battle to fight against cancer in all frontiers.

6. <u>CONCLUSION:</u>

A number of clinical observations have provided evidence supporting the notion of tumour immune surveillance in humans. The increased risk of tumour development in immunosuppressed patients, instances of spontaneous tumour regression, and the appearance of tumour reactive T cells and B cells in relation to improved prognosis all point to a role for the immune system in suppressing tumour growth. (Swann Jeremy). The recent development of sophisticated tumour models using genetically altered mice and function-blocking monoclonal antibodies has made possible the critical experiments that not only resolved the long-standing controversy surrounding the cancer immunosurveillance hypothesis of Burnet and Thomas but also led to its refinement into the cancer immunoediting hypothesis.[4]

By gaining an improved understanding of the cellular and molecular processes that lead to immunologic tumour rejection in the elimination phase, it will be possible to identify which immune forces need to be augmented to facilitate natural protection against tumours of different tissue origins. By studying the equilibrium phase, it will be possible to understand the genetic processes that lead to development of tumours with reduced immunogenicities and identify the molecular targets of the cancer immunoediting process in order to gain insight into how tumour sculpting can be prevented by stabilizing tumour cell genomes. Finally, by elucidating how tumours escape immune detection and elimination, it will be possible to develop methods to determine the extent to which a tumour has been edited and devise molecular strategies to reverse these cloaking mechanisms and thus unmask tumour immunogenicity.

The tumour microenvironment represents a complex system in which individual immune cells make potentially interconnected decisions to attack tumour cells, ignore their presence, or enhance their development and/or survival.[15]

Immunotherapy is potentially synergistic with other treatment modalities, and approaches that trigger tumour cell death, alter the tumour microenvironment, reduce tolerogenic mechanisms, and stimulate immune responses might act in concert. An improved understanding of the immunobiology of cancer immunoediting and a molecular definition of how tumours are shaped by this process will undoubtedly bring us closer to a more effective use of immunotherapy together with other conventional cancer treatments to prevent, control, and/or eradicate established cancer.[12]

7. BIBLIOGRAPHY:

1. Kumar, Abbas, Fausto, Mitchell, Robbins Basic Pathology, 8th Edition, published by Saunders: An imprint of Elsevier. 2010.

2. Kast MW, Schreiber H, and Velders MP. "Tumour Immunology". EncyclopediaOf Life Sciences 2001; 1-8.

3. Smyth MJ, Godfrey DI, and Trapani A. "A Fresh Look at Tumour Immunosurveillance and Immunotherapy". Nature Immunology 2001 April; 2(4): 293-9.

4. Dunn GP, Old LJ, and Schreiber RD. "The Three Es of Cancer Immunoediting". Annual. Reviews Immunology. 2004; 22:329–60.

5. Igney FH, Krammer PH. "Immune Escape of Tumours: Apoptosis Resistance and Tumour Counterattack" Journal of Leukocyte Biology 2002 June; (71):907-20.

6. Mlecknik B. "Database for Cancer immunology". Master Thesis, Graz University of Technology, 2003.

7. Sudhakar A. "History of Cancer, Ancient and Modern Treatment Methods". J Cancer Sci Ther. 2009 December; 1:1(2)

8. Vanneman M, Dranoff G. "Combining Immunotherapy and targeted therapies in cancer treatment". Nature Review Cancer. 2012 April; 12: 237-51.

9. J. Copier et al. "Improving the efficacy of Cancer Immunotherapy". European Journal of Cancer 2009; 45: 1424-31.

10. Timothy Lee Al. "Immunology for 1st year Medical Students", 3rd ed. Faculty of Medicine, Dalhousie Universit0y 2009.

11. David, Jonathan, David, Ivan. Immunology, 7th Edition, published by Mosby: An imprint of Elsevier. 2007.

12. Swann JB, Smyth MJ. "Immune surveillance of tumours". The Journal of Clinical Investigation.2007 May; 117(5):1137-46.

13. Pradeu T, Cooper EL. "The Danger Theory: 20 years later". Frontiers in Immunology. 2012 September; 3:1-9.

14. Kim R, Emi M, Tanabe K. "Cancer immunoediting from immune surveillance to immune escape". Immunology 2007; 121: 1-14.

15. Bui JD, Schreiber RD. "Cancer immunosurveillance, immunoediting and inflammation: independent or interdependent processes?" Current Opinion in Immunology 2007; 19:203-8.

16. Matzinger P, Fuchs EJ. "Is cancer dangerous to immune system?"Seminars in Immunology, 1996; 8:271-80.

17. Prendergast GC, Jaffee EM. Cancer immunotherapy: Immune suppression and Tumour Growth, 2nd Edition, Academic Press: An imprint of Elsevier 2007.

18. American Cancer Society. "Immunotherapy". 2013.

19. Vivier E, Ugolini S, Blaise D, Chabannon C, Brossay L. Nature Reviews Immunology. 2012 April; 12:239-52.

20. Seung, S, Urban JL, Schreiber H. "A tumour escape variant that has lost one major histocompatibility complex class I restriction element induces specific CD8_ T cells to an antigen that no longer serves as a target." Journal of Experimental Medicine. 1993; 178:933–40.

21. Ranges GE, Figari IS, Espevik, T, Palladino Jr. MA. "Inhibition of cytotoxic T cell development by transforming growth factor beta and reversal by recombinant tumour necrosis factor alpha" Journal of Experimental Medicine. 1987; 166:991–8.

22. Ganss R, Limmer A, Sacher T, Arnold B, Hammerling GJ. "Auto aggression and tumour rejection: it takes more than self-specific T-cell activation." Immunology Review. 1993; 169:263–272.

23. Walker PR, Saas P, Dietrich PY. "Tumour expression of Fas ligand (CD95L) and the consequences." Current Opinion Immunology. 1998; 10:564–72.

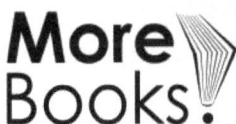
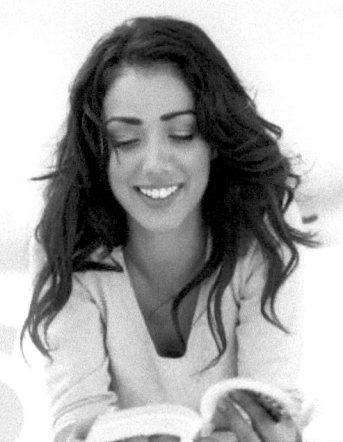

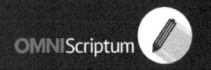

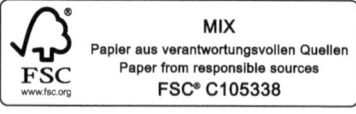
Printed by Books on Demand GmbH, Norderstedt / Germany